RENAL DIET COOKBOOK FOR BEGINNERS

Mastering Kidney-Friendly Cooking with Easy, Flavorful Low-Sodium, Low-Potassium and Low-Phosphorus Recipes! Includes a Step-by-Step 30-Day Meal Planner

Marcel Brandt

IMPORTANT !!!

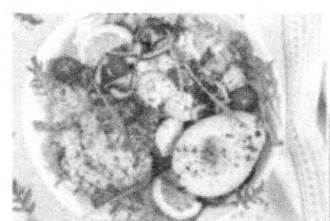

2025

BONUS: The Top Guide for Perfect Renal Portions!

BONUS within the book

SCAN the QR CODE
to Download it

Table of Contents

Introduction

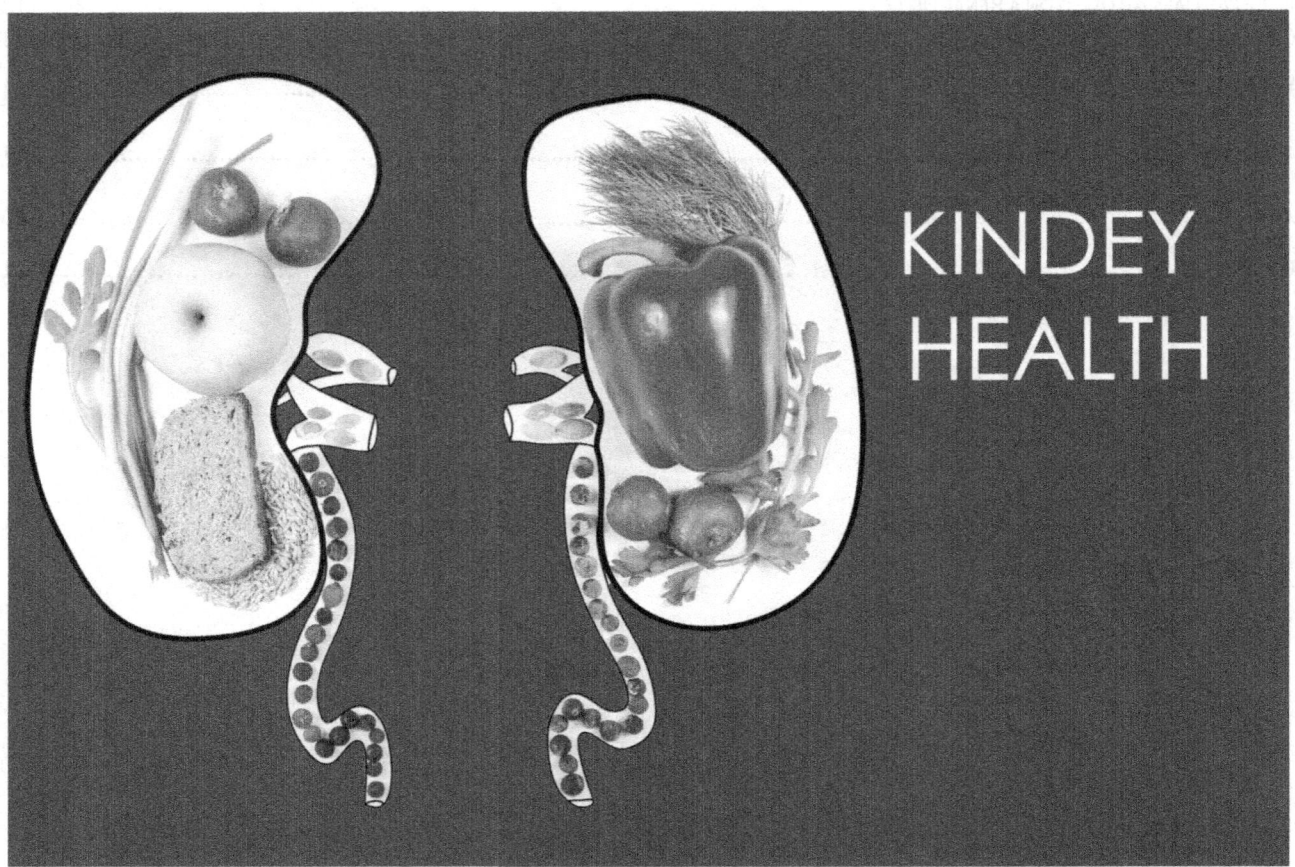

Welcome to the "Renal Diet Cookbook for Beginners," a comprehensive guide to promoting kidney health through mindful and delicious nutrition. This cookbook is designed to support individuals on a renal diet journey, providing a diverse array of flavorful recipes that adhere to the specific dietary requirements essential for maintaining optimal kidney function.

Brief Presentation and Purpose

The purpose of this cookbook is to empower individuals with kidney-related concerns by offering a range of recipes that not only cater to their dietary needs but also celebrate the joy of eating. Each dish has been carefully crafted to strike a balance between nutrition and taste, ensuring that following a renal diet doesn't mean sacrificing flavor or variety.

Inside, you'll find a wealth of information about renal-friendly ingredients, cooking techniques, and meal plans tailored to support kidney health. Whether you're a beginner in the realm of renal diets or seeking fresh inspiration for your culinary repertoire, this cookbook is here to guide you on a flavorful and health-conscious journey.

The Importance of a Renal Diet for Kidney Health

The kidneys play a crucial role in maintaining the body's internal balance by filtering waste and excess fluids from the blood, regulating electrolytes, and producing hormones. A renal diet is specifically designed to lighten the workload on the kidneys, supporting their function and potentially slowing the progression of kidney-related conditions.

Managing nutrient intake, especially monitoring protein, sodium, potassium, and phosphorus levels, is vital for individuals with compromised kidney function. This cookbook takes the guesswork out of meal planning, offering recipes that are not only appetizing but also mindful of these essential nutritional considerations.

Who Should Follow a Renal Diet

A renal diet is beneficial for individuals facing various kidney-related challenges, including those diagnosed with chronic kidney disease (CKD), kidney stones, or other renal disorders. Additionally, individuals at risk of developing kidney problems, such as those with diabetes or high blood pressure, can also benefit from adopting a renal-friendly eating plan.

Whether you are navigating the complexities of managing an existing kidney condition or taking proactive steps to safeguard your kidney health, this cookbook is a valuable resource. With a focus on culinary creativity and nutritional awareness, it provides a roadmap for transforming everyday meals into kidney-friendly delights.

Embark on this culinary journey with us, as we explore the intersection of health and flavor, proving that a renal diet can be both nourishing and delightful. Your path to better kidney health starts in your kitchen, and we're here to make it a journey filled with delicious possibilities.

Chapter 1: What is the Renal Diet?

The term "renal diet" refers to a specialized eating plan designed to promote kidney health and manage various kidney conditions. This dietary approach is crucial for individuals with kidney diseases, as it helps alleviate symptoms, slow down the progression of the disease, and maintain overall well-being. A renal diet is typically prescribed by healthcare professionals, including nephrologists and dietitians, based on an individual's specific kidney function, medical history, and nutritional needs.

What is a Renal Diet?

A renal diet is primarily focused on regulating the intake of certain nutrients to ease the workload on the kidneys. The kidneys play a vital role in filtering waste products and excess fluids from the blood, maintaining a balance of electrolytes, and regulating blood pressure. When kidneys are impaired due to disease or other conditions, adjustments in the diet become essential to support kidney function and prevent complications.

Benefits of a Renal Diet

The benefits of adhering to a renal diet are multifaceted. First and foremost, it helps manage the symptoms of kidney disease, such as fluid retention, electrolyte imbalances, and high blood pressure. Additionally, a renal diet aids in preserving the remaining kidney function and slows down the progression of kidney disease. It can also minimize the risk of complications associated with impaired kidney function, such as cardiovascular disease.

Foods to Include and Avoid in a Renal Diet

Foods to Include:

Low-Potassium Foods: Potassium is a mineral that needs to be regulated in a renal diet. Foods low in potassium include apples, berries, cabbage, and green beans.

Low-Phosphorus Foods: Phosphorus balance is critical for kidney health. Individuals on a renal diet may limit phosphorus intake by choosing low-phosphorus foods such as rice, pasta, and certain fruits and vegetables.

Low-Sodium Foods: Sodium can contribute to fluid retention and high blood pressure. A renal diet typically involves reducing sodium intake by choosing fresh fruits and vegetables, using herbs and spices for flavor, and avoiding processed foods.

Lean Proteins: High-quality protein sources like poultry, fish, and eggs are preferred over red meats. This helps minimize the burden on the kidneys while still meeting the body's protein needs.

Foods to Avoid:

High-Potassium Foods: Bananas, oranges, tomatoes, and potatoes are examples of foods rich in potassium that individuals with kidney disease may need to limit.

High-Phosphorus Foods: Dairy products, nuts, and seeds are high in phosphorus and may be restricted in a renal diet.

High-Sodium Foods: Processed and canned foods, as well as certain condiments, are often high in sodium and should be limited or avoided.

How a Renal Diet Helps in the Management of Kidney Diseases

A renal diet plays a pivotal role in managing kidney diseases by addressing specific nutritional needs and mitigating stress on the kidneys. Here's how it contributes to the overall management:

Maintaining Fluid Balance: Proper fluid intake helps manage fluid retention, a common issue in kidney diseases. Monitoring and restricting fluid intake are essential aspects of a renal diet.

Managing Electrolyte Levels: Regulating potassium, phosphorus, and sodium intake helps maintain the balance of electrolytes in the body, preventing complications such as electrolyte imbalances and bone disorders.

Preserving Kidney Function: By reducing the workload on the kidneys, a renal diet aims to preserve the remaining kidney function and slow down the progression of kidney disease.

Supporting Cardiovascular Health: Since kidney diseases often coexist with cardiovascular issues, a renal diet, which includes heart-healthy choices, contributes to overall cardiovascular well-being.

In conclusion, a renal diet is a crucial component of kidney disease management, tailored to individual needs to optimize nutrition while minimizing stress on the kidneys. It empowers individuals to take an active role in their health and work collaboratively with healthcare professionals for the best possible outcomes.

Chapter 2: Basic Principles of the Renal Diet for Beginners

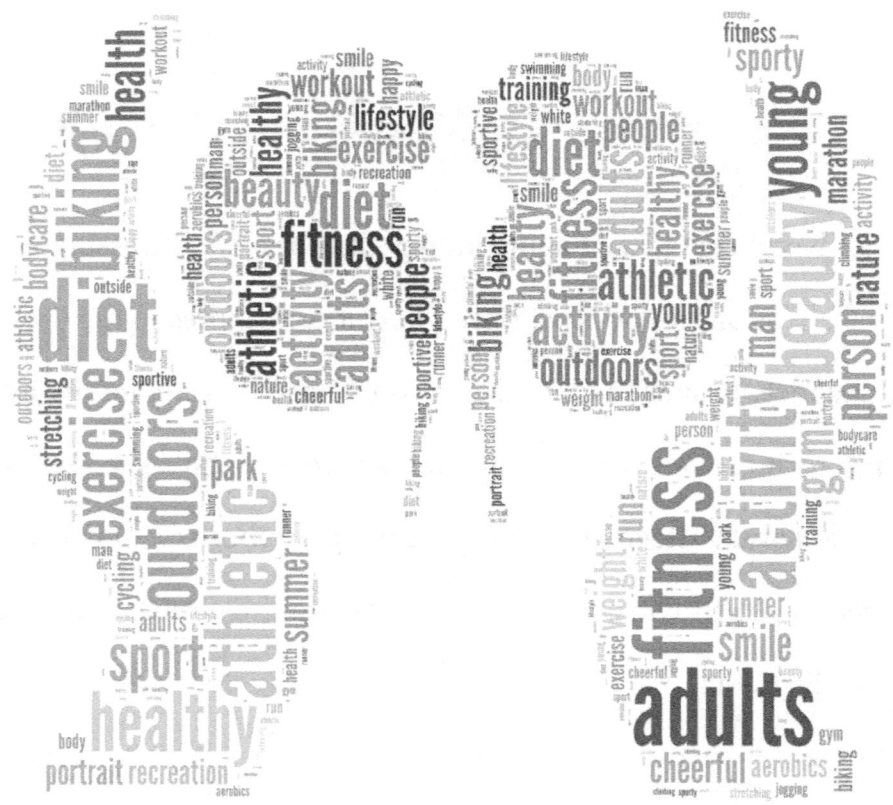

The renal diet is a crucial aspect of managing kidney health for individuals with kidney disease. This specialized diet focuses on maintaining optimal kidney function by regulating the intake of certain nutrients. Understanding the basic principles of the renal diet is essential for beginners to effectively manage their condition and improve overall well-being.

Balancing Fluid Intake:

One of the fundamental principles of the renal diet is maintaining an appropriate fluid balance. Individuals with kidney disease often experience difficulty in regulating fluid levels, leading to complications. Monitoring fluid intake is crucial to avoid fluid retention and swelling. This involves not only monitoring beverages but also considering the fluid content in various foods like fruits and soups.

Controlling Sodium Intake

Sodium plays a significant role in fluid balance and blood pressure regulation. A key aspect of the renal diet is limiting sodium intake to prevent hypertension and fluid retention. This involves minimizing the consumption of processed and packaged foods, as they often contain high levels of sodium. Fresh, whole foods and herbs can be used to enhance flavor without compromising on health.

Managing Protein Intake

Protein is an essential component of a healthy diet, but excessive protein intake can strain the kidneys. The renal diet focuses on moderating protein consumption, especially for those with advanced kidney disease.

High-quality protein sources like lean meats, fish, eggs, and plant-based proteins are preferred, while processed and red meats should be limited.

Watching Potassium and Phosphorus

Another crucial element of the renal diet involves monitoring potassium and phosphorus levels. Kidneys play a role in regulating these minerals, and imbalances can lead to complications. Foods rich in potassium, such as bananas and oranges, should be consumed in moderation. Similarly, phosphorus-rich foods like dairy products and nuts should be controlled.

Limiting Oxalate Intake

For some individuals with kidney stones or specific kidney conditions, limiting foods high in oxalates is important. Oxalates can contribute to the formation of kidney stones, so reducing the intake of foods like spinach, beets, and nuts can be beneficial.

Guide to Meal Planning and Nutrient Balancing

Effective meal planning is at the core of a successful renal diet. Focus on creating well-balanced meals that include a variety of nutrient-dense foods. Distribute protein, carbohydrates, and fats evenly throughout the day, and incorporate a mix of colorful fruits and vegetables. Working with a dietitian can help tailor a meal plan to individual needs and preferences.

Tips on How to Read Food Labels and Make Conscious Choices

Learning to decipher food labels is crucial in making informed choices. Pay attention to sodium, potassium, and phosphorus content. Choose low-sodium alternatives, opt for fresh or frozen produce, and be cautious of hidden additives. Being conscious of portion sizes and monitoring nutritional information empowers individuals to make kidney-friendly choices.

Adapting the Renal Diet to Everyday Life

Successfully integrating the renal diet into everyday life involves practical considerations. Plan meals ahead, carry snacks, and communicate dietary needs to friends and family. Social events and dining out can still be enjoyable with careful choices. Flexibility and creativity in the kitchen make the renal diet sustainable and enjoyable.

Shopping List - What to Eat and What to Avoid

Creating a renal-friendly shopping list is a key component of the diet. Include items like fresh fruits, vegetables, lean meats, fish, eggs, and whole grains. Conversely, limit or avoid processed foods, high-sodium items, and those rich in phosphorus and potassium. Being mindful while grocery shopping sets the stage for successful adherence to the renal diet.

A renal diet, also known as a kidney-friendly diet, is designed to help individuals with kidney disease manage their condition by reducing the intake of certain nutrients that the kidneys may have difficulty processing. It's important to consult with a healthcare professional or a registered dietitian to create a personalized renal diet plan based on individual health needs. However, here is a general guideline for a renal diet, including foods to eat and foods to avoid:

Foods to Eat on a Renal Diet:

Low-Potassium Fruits:

Apples

Berries (strawberries, blueberries, raspberries)

Pineapple (in moderation)

Watermelon (in moderation)

Low-Phosphorus Vegetables:

Bell peppers

Cabbage

Cauliflower

Green beans

Kale

Onions

Lean Proteins:

Skinless poultry

Fish (low in phosphorus, such as salmon, trout, and tuna)

Eggs

Lean cuts of beef or pork

Low-Sodium Foods:

Fresh herbs and spices for flavoring instead of salt

Low-sodium broths

Fresh vegetables

Grains and Starches:

White bread

White rice

Pasta

Cereals with low phosphorus and potassium content

Dairy Alternatives:

Unenriched rice milk

Almond milk (low phosphorus)

Low-phosphorus cheeses

Healthy Fats:

Olive oil

Canola oil

Avocado (in moderation)

Desserts (in moderation):

Sorbet

Sherbet

Angel food cake

Foods to Avoid on a Renal Diet

High-Potassium Foods:

Bananas

Oranges

Potatoes

Tomatoes

Avocados

High-Phosphorus Foods:

Dairy products (milk, cheese, yogurt)

Nuts and seeds

Chocolate

Whole grains

High-Sodium Foods:

Processed foods

Canned soups and broths

Deli meats

Pickles

Limit Phosphorus Additives:

Check food labels for phosphorus additives (look for words with "phos" in them)

Limit Fluid Intake:

Depending on individual needs, fluid intake may need to be restricted. This includes water, juice, and other beverages.

Limit Potassium and Phosphorus Binders:

Some individuals may need medications or binders to help control potassium and phosphorus levels.

Remember, it's crucial to tailor the diet to individual needs and medical conditions. Regular monitoring and adjustments to the diet plan by a healthcare professional are essential for those with kidney disease.

Chapter 3: Preparing for the Renal Diet

Living with kidney disease requires careful attention to dietary choices to manage the health of your kidneys. A crucial aspect of this management is adopting a renal diet, which aims to reduce the burden on your kidneys while providing essential nutrients. In this chapter, we will explore the necessary steps to prepare for a renal diet, including tips for shopping and choosing ingredients, essential kitchen tools for meal preparation, and advice on storing and organizing foods.

Tips for Shopping and Choosing Ingredients

Fresh is Best: Prioritize fresh produce, lean proteins, and whole grains. Choose fruits and vegetables with vibrant colors, as they are rich in essential vitamins and minerals.

Mindful Meat Selection: Opt for lean proteins such as poultry, fish, and lean cuts of meat. Remove excess skin and fat before cooking, as these can contribute to higher phosphorus and sodium levels.

Read Labels: Familiarize yourself with food labels to identify phosphorus and sodium content. Choose low-phosphorus and low-sodium options whenever possible.

Limit Processed Foods: Processed and convenience foods often contain hidden additives, sodium, and phosphorus. Minimize their consumption to better control your nutrient intake.

Control Potassium Intake: Choose lower-potassium fruits and vegetables, such as apples, berries, and green beans. Be cautious with high-potassium foods like bananas, oranges, and tomatoes, and monitor your intake accordingly.

Plan Meals Ahead: Create a weekly meal plan and shopping list to stay organized. This can help you make healthier choices and avoid impulsive purchases that may not align with your renal diet.

Essential Kitchen Tools for Meal Preparation

Food Scale: Precise measurements are crucial in managing nutrient intake. A food scale helps you control portion sizes and adhere to dietary guidelines.

Quality Knives: Invest in sharp, high-quality knives for efficient and safe food preparation. This is particularly important when cutting fruits, vegetables, and lean meats.

Nonstick Cookware: Using nonstick pans reduces the need for excessive oil and makes cooking and cleaning easier. This promotes healthier cooking methods for individuals on a renal diet.

Blender or Food Processor: These tools are essential for creating smoothies, purees, and sauces. They are especially useful for individuals who may have difficulty chewing or swallowing certain foods.

Steamer Basket: Steaming is a kidney-friendly cooking method that helps retain nutrients while minimizing the need for added fats. A steamer basket is a versatile tool for cooking vegetables, fish, and other renal-friendly foods.

Advice on Storing and Organizing Foods

Label and Date: Clearly label and date leftovers and pre-prepared meals to ensure freshness and avoid consuming items beyond their recommended storage period.

Portion Control: Use portion-sized containers to divide meals into appropriate serving sizes. This can help you avoid overeating and ensure consistent nutrient intake.

Freezer-Friendly Options: Prepare and freeze renal-friendly meals in advance. This not only saves time but also ensures you always have suitable options available.

Organize the Fridge: Keep kidney-friendly foods at eye level in the refrigerator for easy access. This visual reminder can help you make healthier choices when reaching for a snack or preparing a meal.

By adopting these tips and incorporating the right tools into your kitchen, you'll be better equipped to navigate the challenges of a renal diet and support the health of your kidneys. Remember, consulting with a healthcare professional or a registered dietitian is essential to tailor dietary recommendations to your specific needs and condition.

Chapter 4: Renal Diet Recipes

Breakfast

1. Quick Berry Blast Smoothie

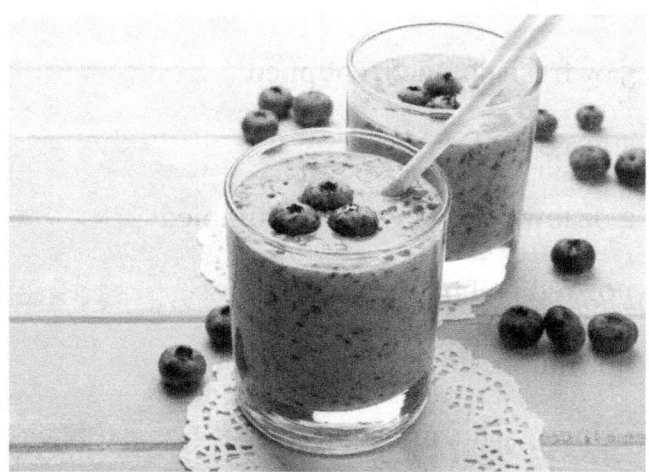

Preparation Time: 5 mins | Cooking Time: 0 mins | Serving Size: 2

Ingredients:

5 oz mixed berries (strawberries, blueberries, raspberries)

7 oz low-potassium Greek yogurt

3.5 oz ice cubes

2 tsp chia seeds

1 tsp honey (optional)

2/3 cup water

Instructions:

In a blender, combine the mixed berries, low-potassium Greek yogurt, ice cubes, chia seeds, and water.

Blend the ingredients on high speed until the mixture is smooth and well combined.

Taste the smoothie and add honey if desired. Blend again to incorporate the honey.

Pour the smoothie into glasses and serve immediately.

Nutrition (Per serving): Calories 150 | Fat 4g | Carbs 20g | Protein 8g

2. Easy Banana Almond Porridge

Preparation Time: 10 mins | Cooking Time: 10 mins | Serving Size: 2

Ingredients:

1 cup steel-cut oats

1 1/4 cups water

3/4 cup unsweetened almond milk

1 ripe banana, mashed

1 oz chopped almonds

1/2 tsp ground cinnamon

1/2 tsp vanilla extract

A pinch of salt

Instructions:

In a medium-sized saucepan, combine water, almond milk, and salt. Bring it to a gentle boil.

Stir in the steel-cut oats and reduce the heat to low. Let it simmer for 8-10 mins, stirring occasionally.

Once the oats are creamy and cooked to your liking, add the mashed banana, chopped almonds, ground cinnamon, and vanilla extract. Mix well.

Continue cooking for an additional 2-3 mins until the banana is fully incorporated, and the porridge reaches your desired consistency.

Remove the saucepan from heat and let the porridge sit for a minute.

Serve the banana almond porridge in bowls, and if desired, top with additional banana slices and a sprinkle of chopped almonds.

Nutrition (Per Serving): Calories 350 | Fat 12g | Carbs 50g | Protein 10g

3. Protein-Packed Spinach Omelette

Preparation Time: 10 mins | Cooking Time: 10 mins | Serving Size: 2

Ingredients:

5 oz fresh spinach, chopped

4 large eggs

2 oz low-fat feta cheese, crumbled

1 oz red bell pepper, diced

1 oz onion, finely chopped

1 clove garlic, minced

1 tsp olive oil

Salt and pepper to taste

Instructions:

Prepare Ingredients:

Wash and chop the fresh spinach.

Crumble the low-fat feta cheese.

Dice the red bell pepper and finely chop the onion.

Mince the garlic.

Saute Vegetables:

Heat olive oil in a non-stick pan over medium heat.

Add diced red bell pepper, chopped onion, and minced garlic. Saute until the vegetables are tender.

Add Spinach:

Add the chopped spinach to the pan and cook until wilted. Remove any excess liquid.

Whisk Eggs:

In a bowl, whisk the eggs until well beaten.

Combine Ingredients:

Pour the beaten eggs over the sauteed vegetables.

Sprinkle crumbled feta cheese evenly over the eggs.

Cook Omelette:

Cook the omelette on medium heat until the edges set, then gently lift them to let the uncooked eggs flow underneath.

Continue cooking until the omelette is set but still moist on top.

Fold and Serve:

Carefully fold the omelette in half using a spatula.

Slide it onto a plate and season with salt and pepper to taste.

Nutrition (Per Serving): Calories 280 | Fat 18g | Carbs 9g | Protein 21g

4. Wholesome Blueberry Pancakes

Preparation Time: 15 mins | Cooking Time: 15 mins | Serving Size: 4 persons

Ingredients:

1 3/4 cups whole wheat flour

2 tsp baking powder

1 tsp sugar

1/2 tsp salt

9 oz fresh blueberries

2 large eggs

1 cup low-fat milk

2 tbsp unsalted butter, melted

Cooking spray or additional butter for the pan

Instructions:

In a large mixing bowl, combine the whole wheat flour, baking powder, sugar, and salt.

In a separate bowl, whisk together the eggs, low-fat milk, and melted butter.

Pour the wet ingredients into the dry ingredients, stirring until just combined. Be careful not to overmix; a few lumps are okay. Gently fold in the fresh blueberries.

Heat a non-stick skillet or griddle over medium heat. Lightly coat with cooking spray or butter.

Pour 1/4 cup of batter onto the skillet for each pancake. Cook until bubbles form on the surface, then flip and cook until golden brown on the other side.

Repeat until all the batter is used.

Serve the blueberry pancakes warm, topped with additional blueberries or a dollop of low-fat yogurt if desired.

Nutrition (Per serving): Calories 230 | Fat 6g | Carbs 38g | Protein 8g

5. Speedy Mango Tango Smoothie

Preparation Time: 5 mins | Cooking Time: 0 mins | Serving Size: 2

Ingredients:

1 cup mixed berries (strawberries, blueberries, raspberries) - lower in potassium compared to mango

1 cup low-fat Greek yogurt

1 cup ice cubes

2 tbsp chia seeds

1 tsp honey (optional)

2/3 cup water

Instructions:

In a blender, combine the mixed berries, low-fat Greek yogurt, ice cubes, chia seeds, and water.

Blend on high speed until the mixture is smooth.

Taste the smoothie and, if desired, add honey for sweetness. Blend again to incorporate.

Pour into glasses and serve immediately.

Nutrition (Per serving): Calories: 156 | Fat: 7 g | Carbs: 9 g | Protein: 3 g

6. Simple Cinnamon Apple Porridge

Preparation Time: 10 mins | Cooking Time: 15 mins | Serving Size: 2

Ingredients:

1 cup steel-cut oats

10.5 oz apples, peeled, cored, and diced

2 tsp unsalted butter

1 tsp ground cinnamon

1 tbsp honey (optional)

2 cups water

1 cup low-fat milk

A pinch of salt

Instructions:

Prepare Ingredients:

Measure 100g of steel-cut oats.

Peel, core, and dice 300g of apples.

Gather 10g of unsalted butter, 1 tsp of ground cinnamon, 1 tbsp of honey (optional), 500ml of water, 250ml of low-fat milk, and a pinch of salt.

Cooking:

In a medium-sized pot, bring 500ml of water to a boil.

Add the steel-cut oats to the boiling water and stir. Reduce heat to low and simmer for 10 mins, stirring occasionally.

Prepare Apples:

In a separate pan, melt the unsalted butter over medium heat.

Add the diced apples and cook until they are tender but not mushy, approximately 5 mins.

Sprinkle ground cinnamon over the apples and stir well.

Combine Oats and Apples:

Add the cooked apples to the simmering oats.

Pour in 250ml of low-fat milk and stir gently.

Continue simmering for an additional 5 mins or until the oats reach your desired consistency.

Sweeten (Optional):

If desired, add honey for sweetness and stir until well combined.

Serve:

Divide the cinnamon apple porridge into two

.

Nutrition (Per Serving): Calories 300 | Fat 6g | Carbs 55g | Protein 8g

7. High-Protein Veggie Omelette Cups

Preparation Time: 15 mins | Cooking Time: 20 mins | Serving Size: 2

Ingredients:

5 oz cherry tomatoes, diced

3.5 oz spinach, chopped

2.8 oz bell peppers, finely diced

1.8 oz red onion, minced

5.3 oz mushrooms, sliced

4 oz feta cheese, crumbled

8 large eggs

2 tbsp low-fat milk

Salt and pepper to taste

Instructions:

Preheat the Oven: Preheat your oven to 180°C (356°F).

Prepare Veggies: In a non-stick skillet over medium heat, sauté the cherry tomatoes, spinach, bell peppers, red onion, and mushrooms until tender. Set aside.

Whisk Eggs: In a large bowl, whisk together eggs, milk, salt, and pepper until well combined.

Combine Ingredients: Add the sautéed vegetables and crumbled feta to the egg mixture. Mix thoroughly.

Prepare Muffin Tin: Lightly grease a muffin tin with cooking spray.

Fill Muffin Cups: Pour the egg and vegetable mixture evenly into the muffin cups.

Bake: Bake in the preheated oven for 15-20 mins or until the eggs are set.

Serve: Allow the omelette cups to cool for a few mins before removing them from the muffin tin. Serve warm.

Nutrition (Per serving): Calories 280 | Fat 18g | Carbs 10g | Protein 20g

8. Nutty Banana Walnut Muffins

Preparation Time: 15 mins | Cooking Time: 25 mins | Serving Size: 4

Ingredients:

1 cup ripe apples, mashed

1 cup whole wheat flour

1/2 cup oat flour

1/4 cup chopped walnuts

3 tbsp unsalted butter, melted

3 tbsp honey

1 large egg

1 tsp baking powder

1/2 tsp baking soda

1/4 tsp salt

1/2 tsp cinnamon

1/4 tsp nutmeg

1/2 cup low-fat yogurt

Instructions:

Preheat the oven to 350°F (175°C). Line a muffin tin with paper liners.

In a large bowl, mix the mashed apples, melted butter, honey, egg, and yogurt.

In another bowl, combine whole wheat flour, oat flour, baking powder, baking soda, salt, cinnamon, and nutmeg.

Gradually mix the dry ingredients into the wet ingredients until just combined.

Fold in the chopped walnuts.

Fill the muffin cups two-thirds full with batter.

Bake for 20-25 mins, or until a toothpick comes out clean.

Cool in the tin for 5 mins, then transfer to a wire rack.

Nutrition (Per Serving): Calories 250 | Fat 10g | Carbs 35g | Protein 6g

9. Refreshing Green Smoothie

Preparation Time: 10 mins | Cooking Time: 0 mins | Serving Size: 2

Ingredients:

1 cup fresh spinach leaves

4 oz cucumber, peeled and sliced

2 oz celery, chopped

1 small green apple, cored and diced (approx. 4 oz)

1/2 ripe avocado, peeled and pitted

1 cup cold water

2 tbsp fresh lemon juice

Ice cubes (optional)

Instructions:

Prepare the ingredients: rinse spinach, peel and slice cucumber, chop celery, dice apple, and pit avocado.

In a blender, combine spinach, cucumber, celery, apple, and avocado.

Add cold water and lemon juice for a refreshing zest.

Blend until smooth. If desired, add ice for a colder texture.

Serve the citrus green smoothie immediately.

Nutrition (Per Serving): Calories: 167 | Fat: 12 g | Carbs: 7 g | Protein: 9 g

10. Creamy Coconut Chia Porridge

Preparation Time: 10 mins | Cooking Time: 0 mins | Serving Size: 2

Ingredients:

1/3 cup chia seeds

3/4 cup unsweetened coconut milk

2/3 cup water

1/3 oz unsweetened shredded coconut

1 tsp erythritol (or preferred sugar substitute)

1/4 tsp vanilla extract

A pinch of salt

Fresh berries for topping (optional)

Instructions:

In a mixing bowl, combine chia seeds, coconut milk, water, shredded coconut, erythritol, vanilla extract, and a pinch of salt.

Stir the mixture thoroughly to ensure that the chia seeds are evenly distributed.

Let the mixture sit for about 5 mins, stirring occasionally to prevent clumping.

After 5 mins, cover the bowl and refrigerate for at least 4 hours or overnight. This allows the chia seeds to absorb the liquid and create a creamy texture.

Before serving, give the porridge a good stir. If it's too thick, you can add a bit more coconut milk or water to reach your desired consistency.

Divide the creamy coconut chia porridge into two portions.

Top with fresh berries if desired.

Nutrition (Per Serving): Calories 280 | Fat 18g | Carbs 20g | Protein 7g

11. Lean Turkey and Veggie Omelette

Preparation Time: 15 mins | Cooking Time: 10 mins | Serving Size: 2

Ingredients:

5 oz lean ground turkey

3.5 oz bell peppers, diced

2.6 oz cherry tomatoes, halved

1.8 oz spinach, chopped

4 large eggs

1 oz low-fat feta cheese, crumbled

2 tsp olive oil

Salt and pepper to taste

Instructions:

In a non-stick skillet, heat olive oil over medium heat.

Add lean ground turkey and cook until browned, breaking it apart with a spatula.

Stir in diced bell peppers and cook until softened.

Add cherry tomatoes and chopped spinach, cooking until spinach wilts and tomatoes are slightly softened.

In a bowl, beat the eggs and season with salt and pepper.

Pour the beaten eggs over the turkey and veggie mixture in the skillet.

Allow the eggs to set slightly, then gently lift the edges with a spatula, letting the uncooked eggs flow underneath.

Once the omelette is mostly set but still slightly runny on top, sprinkle crumbled feta cheese evenly over one half of the omelette.

Carefully fold the other half of the omelette over the cheese-covered half.

Cook for an additional 1-2 mins until the eggs are fully cooked and the cheese is melted.

Nutrition (Per serving): Calories 350 | Fat 20g | Carbs 10g | Protein 30g

12. Quinoa Pancakes with Mixed Berries

Preparation Time: 15 mins | Cooking Time: 15 mins | Serving Size: 4

Ingredients:

1 3/4 cups quinoa flour

2 tsp baking powder

1/2 tsp salt

2 tbsp honey

2 large eggs

1 cup almond milk

1/4 cup melted unsalted butter

1 tsp vanilla extract

5.3 oz mixed berries (strawberries, blueberries, raspberries)

Instructions:

In a large mixing bowl, whisk together quinoa flour, baking powder, and salt.

In a separate bowl, beat the eggs and add honey, almond milk, melted butter, and vanilla extract. Mix well.

Pour the wet ingredients into the dry ingredients, stirring until just combined. Be careful not to overmix; a few lumps are okay. Gently fold in the mixed berries into the batter.

Heat a non-stick skillet or griddle over medium heat. Lightly grease with butter or cooking spray.

Pour 1/4 cup of batter onto the skillet for each pancake. Cook until bubbles form on the surface, then flip and cook the other side until golden brown.

Repeat until all the batter is used.

Nutrition (Per Serving): Calories 320 | Fat 10g | Carbs 50g | Protein 8g

13. Breezy Tropical Smoothie Bowl

Preparation Time: 10 mins | Cooking Time: 0 mins | Serving Size: 2

Ingredients:

7 oz frozen mango chunks

3.5 oz frozen pineapple chunks

5.3 oz Greek yogurt (low-phosphorus)

1 medium banana (sliced, approx. 4 oz)

1 oz unsweetened coconut flakes

2 tbsp chia seeds

1 tbsp flaxseeds

1 tsp honey (optional)

1/2 cup coconut milk (unsweetened)

Instructions:

In a blender, combine the frozen mango chunks, frozen pineapple chunks, Greek yogurt, sliced banana, and coconut milk.

Blend the ingredients until smooth and creamy. If the mixture is too thick, you can add a bit more coconut milk to reach your desired consistency.

Pour the smoothie into two bowls, evenly distributing the mixture.

Toppings: 4. Sprinkle each bowl with unsweetened coconut flakes, chia seeds, and flaxseeds.

Drizzle a tsp of honey on top for added sweetness if desired.

Serve immediately and enjoy your refreshing Breezy Tropical Smoothie Bowl!

Nutrition (Per Serving): Calories 320 | Fat 15g | Carbs 40g | Protein 8g

14. Five-Minute Chocolate Oat Porridge

Preparation Time: 10 mins | Cooking Time: 0 mins | Serving Size: 2

Ingredients:

1 cup rolled oats

3 tbsp unsweetened cocoa powder

1 ripe banana, mashed

1 1/4 cups unsweetened almond milk

2 tbsp chia seeds

2 tsp honey (optional)

A pinch of salt

Fresh berries for garnish

Instructions:

In a medium-sized saucepan, combine the rolled oats, cocoa powder, mashed banana, almond milk, chia seeds, and a pinch of salt.

Place the saucepan over medium heat and stir the mixture continuously.

Cook for approximately 5 mins or until the porridge reaches your desired consistency. Adjust the thickness by adding more almond milk if needed.

If desired, add honey for sweetness and stir until well combined.

Remove the saucepan from heat and let the porridge sit for a minute to thicken.

Divide the chocolate oat porridge into two serving bowls.

Garnish with fresh berries or your favorite toppings.

Nutrition (Per Serving): Calories 250 | Fat 8g | Carbs 40g | Protein 7g

15. Zesty Tomato and Feta Omelette

Preparation Time: 10 mins | Cooking Time: 10 mins | Serving Size: 2

Ingredients:

5.3 oz cherry tomatoes, halved

2 oz feta cheese, crumbled

4 large eggs

1 oz red bell pepper, diced

1 oz green bell pepper, diced

2 tbsp fresh parsley, chopped

1 tsp olive oil

Salt and pepper to taste

Instructions:

In a bowl, whisk the eggs until well combined. Add a pinch of salt and pepper, then set aside.

Heat olive oil in a non-stick skillet over medium heat.

Add diced red and green bell peppers to the skillet. Sauté until they begin to soften, about 2-3 mins.

Add the halved cherry tomatoes to the skillet and cook for an additional 2 mins, allowing them to release their juices.

Pour the whisked eggs over the vegetables in the skillet.

Sprinkle crumbled feta evenly over the eggs.

Allow the omelette to cook undisturbed for a few mins until the edges set.

Using a spatula, gently lift the edges of the omelette, tilting the skillet to let the uncooked eggs flow to the edges.

Once the omelette is mostly set but still slightly runny on top, fold it in half using the spatula.

Continue cooking for another 2-3 mins or until the eggs are fully cooked and the cheese is melted.

Sprinkle chopped fresh parsley over the top for a burst of freshness.

Carefully transfer the omelette to a plate and serve hot.

Nutrition (Per serving): Calories: 167 | Fat: 9 g | Carbs: 12 g | Protein: 17 g

16. Gluten-Free Blueberry Muffins

Preparation Time: 15 mins | Cooking Time: 25 mins | Serving Size: 4

Ingredients:

1 3/4 cups gluten-free all-purpose flour

3.5 oz almond flour

2 tsp baking powder

1 tsp baking soda

1/2 tsp salt

5.3 oz unsalted butter, melted

5.3 oz granulated sugar

2 large eggs

7 oz plain Greek yogurt

1 tsp vanilla extract

7 oz fresh blueberries

Instructions:

Preheat the oven to 180°C (350°F) and line a muffin tin with paper liners.

In a large bowl, whisk together the gluten-free all-purpose flour, almond flour, baking powder, baking soda, and salt.

In another bowl, cream together the melted butter and sugar until well combined.

Add the eggs one at a time, beating well after each addition. Stir in the Greek yogurt and vanilla extract.

Gradually add the dry ingredients to the wet ingredients, mixing until just combined. Be careful not to overmix.

Gently fold in the fresh blueberries until evenly distributed throughout the batter.

Divide the batter evenly among the muffin cups, filling each about 2/3 full.

Bake in the preheated oven for 20-25 mins or until a toothpick inserted into the center of a muffin comes out clean.

Allow the muffins to cool in the tin for 5 mins before transferring them to a wire rack to cool completely.

Nutrition (Per Serving): Calories 320 | Fat 18g | Carbs 35g | Protein 7g

17. Protein-Packed Peanut Butter Smoothie

Preparation Time: 5 mins | Cooking Time: 0 mins | Serving Size: 2

Ingredients:

7 oz (approx. 14 tbsp) frozen banana slices

5 oz (approx. 10 tbsp) unsweetened almond milk

1.75 oz (approx. 3.5 tbsp) Greek yogurt

1 oz (approx. 2 tbsp) smooth peanut butter

2 tsp chia seeds

1 tsp honey (optional)

Ice cubes (optional)

Instructions:

In a blender, combine the frozen banana slices, low-potassium almond milk, low-potassium Greek yogurt, smooth peanut butter, and chia seeds.

If you prefer a sweeter smoothie, add honey to taste (considering dietary restrictions) and blend until smooth.

If you like a thicker consistency, add a few ice cubes and blend again until well combined.

Pour the smoothie into serving glasses.

Serve immediately and enjoy your Protein-Packed Peanut Butter Smoothie!

Nutrition (Per Serving): Calories: 156 | Fat: 7 g | Carbs: 12 g | Protein: 9 g

18. Easy Apple Cinnamon Pancakes

Preparation Time: 15 mins | Cooking Time: 15 mins | Serving Size: 4

Ingredients:

1 3/4 cups all-purpose flour

2 tsp baking powder

1 tsp ground cinnamon

A pinch of salt

1 cup unsweetened applesauce

2 large eggs

2 tbsp unsalted butter, melted

1 tbsp sugar substitute

1 cup low-fat milk

1 medium apple, peeled, cored, and finely diced

Instructions:

In a large mixing bowl, combine the flour, baking powder, cinnamon, and salt.

In another bowl, whisk together the applesauce, eggs, melted butter, and sugar substitute.

Gradually mix the wet ingredients into the dry ingredients until just combined.

Stir in the milk to achieve a smooth batter, then fold in the diced apple.

Heat a non-stick skillet over medium heat and lightly grease with cooking spray.

Pour 1/4 cup of batter for each pancake, cooking until bubbles form on the surface, then flip and cook until golden.

Serve warm with a suitable sugar-free syrup or fresh fruit.

Nutrition (Per serving): Calories 280 | Fat 8g | Carbs 45g | Protein 7g

19. Spinach and Mushroom Egg White Omelette

Preparation Time: 10 mins | Cooking Time: 15 mins | Serving Size: 2

Ingredients:

8.75 oz (approx. 17.5 tbsp) egg whites

1.75 oz (approx. 3.5 tbsp) spinach, chopped

1.75 oz (approx. 3.5 tbsp) mushrooms, sliced

1 oz (approx. 2 tbsp) onion, finely diced

1 clove garlic, minced

1 tsp olive oil

Salt and pepper to taste

Fresh herbs for garnish (optional)

Instructions:

In a non-stick pan, heat olive oil over medium heat.

Add onions and garlic, sauté until translucent.

Add mushrooms and spinach, cook until mushrooms are tender and spinach is wilted.

In a separate bowl, whisk the egg whites until frothy.

Pour the whisked egg whites over the vegetables in the pan.

Allow the eggs to set slightly at the edges, then gently stir the mixture.

Continue cooking, stirring occasionally, until the eggs are fully cooked but still moist.

Season with salt and pepper to taste.

Garnish with fresh herbs if desired.

Serve hot and enjoy your kidney-friendly Spinach and Mushroom Egg White Omelette!

Nutrition (Per Serving): Calories 180 | Fat 6g | Carbs 8g | Protein 24g

20. Sweet Potato Pancakes with Maple Pecan Glaze

Preparation Time: 15 mins | Cooking Time: 15 mins | Serving Size: 4

Ingredients:

2 cups grated zucchini

1 1/2 cups whole wheat flour

2 large eggs

1 cup low-fat milk

1 tsp baking powder

1/2 tsp cinnamon

1/4 tsp nutmeg

A pinch of salt

1 tbsp vegetable oil

Maple Pecan Glaze:

1/4 cup pecans, chopped

1/2 cup sugar-free maple syrup

Instructions:

Squeeze grated zucchini to remove excess moisture. Mix with whole wheat flour, eggs, milk, baking powder, cinnamon, nutmeg, and salt until a smooth batter forms.

Heat oil in a non-stick skillet over medium heat. Spoon 1/4 cup of batter for each pancake, cooking until bubbles form, then flip.

For the glaze, toast pecans in a dry pan, then stir in sugar-free maple syrup and warm through.

Serve pancakes warm, topped with the maple pecan glaze.

Nutrition (Per serving): Calories 320 | Fat 9g | Carbs 54g | Protein 8g

Lunch

21. Quinoa and Veggie Delight Salad

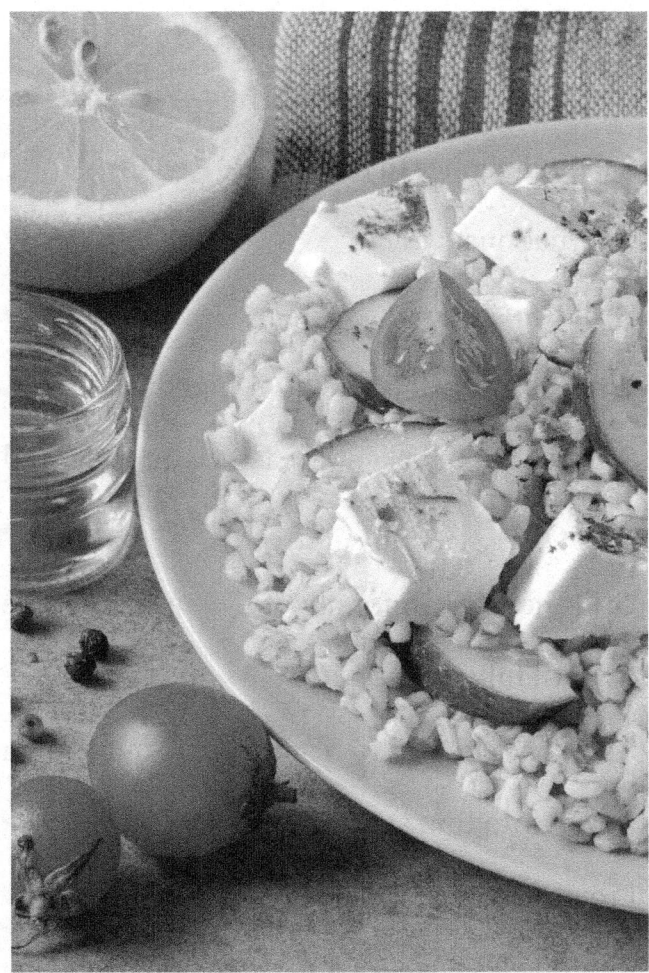

Preparation Time: 15 mins | Cooking Time: 15 mins | Serving Size: 4 portions

Ingredients:

1 cup quinoa, rinsed

14 oz mixed vegetables (carrots, bell peppers, cucumbers), diced

5 oz cherry tomatoes, halved

3.5 oz baby spinach

2.8 oz red onion, finely chopped

2 oz feta cheese, crumbled

2 tbsp fresh parsley, chopped

2 tbsp olive oil

1 tbsp balsamic vinegar

Salt and pepper to taste

Instructions:

Cook Quinoa: In a medium saucepan, combine 400ml water and the rinsed quinoa. Bring to a boil, then reduce the heat, cover, and simmer for 15 mins or until the quinoa is cooked and water is absorbed. Allow it to cool.

Prepare Vegetables: While the quinoa is cooking, dice the mixed vegetables, halve the cherry tomatoes, chop the red onion, and crumble the feta cheese.

Assemble Salad: In a large mixing bowl, combine the cooked quinoa, diced vegetables, cherry tomatoes, baby spinach, red onion, feta cheese, and chopped parsley.

Make Dressing: In a small bowl, whisk together olive oil, balsamic vinegar, salt, and pepper.

Dress the Salad: Pour the dressing over the salad and toss gently until all ingredients are well coated.

Serve: Divide the Quinoa and Veggie Delight Salad into 4 portions.

Nutrition (Per Serving): Calories 350 | Fat 14g | Carbs 45g | Protein 12g

22. Grilled Chicken Caesar Salad with Low-Phosphorus Dressing

Preparation Time: 15 mins | Cooking Time: 15 mins | Serving Size: 4

Ingredients:

14 oz boneless, skinless chicken breasts, grilled and sliced

7 oz romaine lettuce, washed and chopped

3.5 oz cherry tomatoes, halved

1.75 oz Parmesan cheese, shaved

1 tbsp capers, drained

2 tbsp low-phosphorus Caesar dressing

Low-Phosphorus Caesar Dressing:

5.3 oz low-phosphorus mayonnaise

2 tbsp olive oil

1 tbsp lemon juice

2 cloves garlic, minced

1 tsp Dijon mustard

1 tsp anchovy paste

Salt and pepper to taste

Instructions:

Grill the Chicken:

Preheat the grill to medium-high heat.

Season the chicken breasts with salt and pepper.

Grill the chicken for about 6-8 mins per side or until fully cooked.

Allow the chicken to rest for a few mins, then slice it into thin strips.

Prepare the Dressing:

In a bowl, whisk together mayonnaise, olive oil, lemon juice, minced garlic, Dijon mustard, anchovy paste, salt, and pepper until well combined.

Assemble the Salad:

In a large bowl, combine the chopped romaine lettuce, cherry tomatoes, shaved Parmesan cheese, and capers.

Add the grilled chicken slices to the salad.

Dress the Salad:

Drizzle the low-phosphorus Caesar dressing over the salad.

Toss gently to coat the salad evenly with the dressing.

Serve:

Divide the salad among four plates.

Nutrition (Per Serving): Calories 350 | Fat 20g | Carbs 8g | Protein 35g

23. Spinach and Berry Power Salad

Preparation Time: 15 mins | Cooking Time: 0 mins | Serving Size: 4

Ingredients:

7 oz fresh baby spinach leaves

5.3 oz strawberries, hulled and sliced

3.5 oz blueberries

3.5 oz raspberries

1.75 oz almonds, sliced

1 oz feta cheese, crumbled (optional)

1 tbsp chia seeds

For the Dressing:

2 tbsp extra-virgin olive oil

1 tbsp balsamic vinegar

1 tsp honey (optional)

Salt and pepper to taste

Instructions:

Prepare the Salad Base:

Wash the baby spinach leaves thoroughly and pat them dry with a clean kitchen towel.

In a large salad bowl, combine the baby spinach, sliced strawberries, blueberries, raspberries, and almonds.

Make the Dressing:

In a small bowl, whisk together the olive oil, balsamic vinegar, honey (if using), salt, and pepper until well combined.

Assemble the Salad:

Drizzle the dressing over the salad and gently toss to coat the ingredients evenly.

Sprinkle chia seeds on top for an added nutritional boost.

If desired, crumble feta cheese over the salad.

Serve:

Divide the spinach and berry power salad into four equal portions.

Nutrition (Per serving): Calories 180 | Fat 12g | Carbs 15g | Protein 5g

24. Mediterranean Chickpea Salad Bowl

Preparation Time: 15 mins | Cooking Time: 0 mins | Serving Size: 4

Ingredients:

14 oz canned chickpeas, drained and rinsed

7 oz cherry tomatoes, halved

5.3 oz cucumber, diced

3.5 oz red bell pepper, chopped

3.5 oz black olives, sliced

2.8 oz feta cheese, crumbled

2.1 oz red onion, finely chopped

2 tbsp fresh parsley, chopped

For the Dressing:

4 tbsp extra virgin olive oil

2 tbsp red wine vinegar

1 clove garlic, minced

1 tsp dried oregano

Salt and pepper to taste

Instructions:

In a large mixing bowl, combine the chickpeas, cherry tomatoes, cucumber, red bell pepper, black olives, feta cheese, red onion, and fresh parsley.

In a small bowl, whisk together the olive oil, red wine vinegar, minced garlic, dried oregano, salt, and pepper to create the dressing.

Pour the dressing over the salad ingredients and toss gently to coat everything evenly.

Allow the salad to marinate for at least 15 mins to enhance the flavors.

Serve the Mediterranean Chickpea Salad in individual bowls.

Renal Diet Note:

This recipe is suitable for individuals following a renal diet. Monitor portion sizes to ensure adherence to dietary restrictions.

Nutrition (Per Serving): Calories 350 | Fat 20g | Carbs 35g | Protein 10g

25. Roasted Beet and Goat Cheese Salad with Walnuts

Preparation Time: 15 mins | Cooking Time: 30 mins | Serving Size: 4

Ingredients:

4 large carrots, peeled and diced

4 oz goat cheese, crumbled

1/2 cup pecans, chopped

8 oz mixed salad greens

2 tbsp olive oil

1 tbsp balsamic vinegar

Salt and pepper to taste

Instructions:

Preheat the oven to 400°F (200°C).

Toss the diced carrots with 1 tbsp olive oil, salt, and pepper. Spread on a baking sheet.

Roast for 30 mins or until tender and lightly caramelized, stirring halfway through.

Whisk together the remaining olive oil and balsamic vinegar, seasoning with salt and pepper to taste for the dressing.

In a large bowl, combine the roasted carrots, mixed greens, crumbled goat cheese, and pecans.

Drizzle the dressing over the salad, tossing gently to combine.

Serve immediately, adjusting seasoning as needed.

Nutrition (Per serving): Calories 350 | Fat 25g | Carbs 20g | Protein 10g

26. Avocado and Shrimp Citrus Salad

Preparation Time: 15 mins | Cooking Time: 5 mins | Serving Size: 4

Ingredients:

8 oz shrimp, peeled and deveined

1 small avocado, sliced

8 oz mixed salad greens

1 orange, segmented

1/4 cup red onion, thinly sliced

2 tbsp fresh cilantro, chopped

2 tbsp olive oil

1 tbsp lime juice

Salt and pepper to taste

Instructions:

Grill shrimp over medium heat until pink and opaque, about 2-3 mins per side.

In a large bowl, combine salad greens, avocado slices, orange segments, red onion, and cilantro.

Whisk together olive oil, lime juice, salt, and pepper for the dressing.

Add grilled shrimp to the salad. Drizzle with dressing and toss gently.

Serve immediately, offering additional lime wedges if desired.

Nutrition (Per Serving): Calories 350 | Fat 18g | Carbs 25g | Protein 20g

27. Cucumber and Dill Yogurt Salad

Preparation Time: 15 mins | Cooking Time: 0 mins | Serving Size: 4

Ingredients:

1 lb cucumbers, thinly sliced

1 cup Greek yogurt (low-fat)

1 tbsp fresh dill, finely chopped

1 clove garlic, minced

2 tsp white vinegar

Salt and pepper to taste

Instructions:

In a large mixing bowl, combine the Greek yogurt, minced garlic, and white vinegar. Mix well until you achieve a smooth consistency.

Add the thinly sliced cucumbers to the yogurt mixture. Ensure that the cucumbers are evenly coated with the yogurt.

Sprinkle the chopped fresh dill over the cucumbers and yogurt mixture. Mix gently to distribute the dill evenly.

Season the salad with salt and pepper according to your taste preferences. Remember to go easy on the salt, especially for individuals on a renal diet.

Refrigerate the salad for at least 30 mins before serving. This allows the flavors to meld and enhances the overall taste of the dish.

Once chilled, give the salad a final gentle stir before serving. Divide it into four portions.

Nutrition (Per Serving): Calories 80 | Fat 2g | Carbs 8g | Protein 5g

28. Watermelon and Feta Summer Salad

Preparation Time: 15 mins | Cooking Time: 0 mins | Serving Size: 4

Ingredients:

2 large cucumbers, diced

4 oz feta cheese, crumbled

1/2 cup red onion, thinly sliced

1/4 cup fresh mint leaves, chopped

1/4 cup Kalamata olives, pitted and sliced

2 tbsp extra virgin olive oil

1 tbsp balsamic vinegar

Salt and pepper to taste

Instructions:

In a large bowl, combine cucumbers, feta, red onion, mint, and olives.

Whisk together olive oil and balsamic vinegar for the dressing.

Drizzle the dressing over the salad, tossing gently to coat.

Season with salt and pepper, adjusting to taste.

Chill for 15 mins before serving to blend flavors.

Nutrition (Per serving): Calories 210 | Fat 12g | Carbs 22g | Protein 7g

29. Broccoli and Cranberry Almond Salad

Preparation Time: 15 mins | Cooking Time: 2 mins | Serving Size: 4

Ingredients:

1 lb broccoli florets

1/2 cup dried apples, chopped (a lower potassium substitute for cranberries)

1/3 cup sliced almonds

1/2 cup low-fat Greek yogurt

2 tbsp olive oil

1 tbsp apple cider vinegar

1 tsp Dijon mustard

Salt and pepper to taste

Instructions:

Blanch broccoli in boiling water for 2 mins, then plunge into ice water. Drain well.

In a large bowl, combine broccoli, dried apples, and almonds.

Whisk together Greek yogurt, olive oil, vinegar, mustard, salt, and pepper for the dressing.

Toss salad with dressing until evenly coated.

Chill before serving to meld flavors.

Nutrition (Per serving): Calories 250 | Fat 15g | Carbs 25g | Protein 8g

30. Tuna and White Bean Mediterranean Salad

Preparation Time: 15 mins | Cooking Time: 0 mins | Serving Size: 2-4 persons

Ingredients:

1 can (7 oz) tuna in water, drained

2 cups cucumber, diced (substitute for white beans to lower potassium)

1 cup cherry tomatoes, halved

1/2 cup red onion, finely sliced

1/4 cup Kalamata olives, pitted and sliced

2 oz feta cheese, crumbled

2 tbsp fresh parsley, chopped

2 tbsp extra virgin olive oil

1 tbsp red wine vinegar

1 clove garlic, minced

1 tsp dried oregano

Salt and pepper to taste

Instructions:

In a large bowl, combine tuna, cucumbers, cherry tomatoes, red onion, olives, feta, and parsley.

Whisk together olive oil, vinegar, garlic, oregano, salt, and pepper for the dressing.

Pour dressing over salad, tossing gently to coat.

Let salad marinate for 15 mins in the refrigerator before serving.

Nutrition (Per serving): Calories 350 | Fat 15g | Carbs 25g | Protein 28g

31. Lemon Herb Chicken Soup with Brown Rice

Preparation Time: 15 mins | Cooking Time: 40 mins | Serving Size: 4

Ingredients:

1.1 lb boneless, skinless chicken breast, diced

2/3 cup brown rice

1 onion, finely chopped

2 carrots, peeled and diced

2 celery stalks, chopped

3 cloves garlic, minced

1 tbsp olive oil

8 cups low-sodium chicken broth

1 lemon, zest and juice

1 tsp dried thyme

1 tsp dried rosemary

Salt and pepper to taste

- Fresh parsley for garnish

Instructions:

In a large pot, heat olive oil over medium heat. Add onions, carrots, celery, and garlic. Sauté until vegetables are softened, about 5 mins.

Add diced chicken to the pot and cook until browned on all sides.

Pour in the chicken broth, add brown rice, thyme, rosemary, lemon zest, and lemon juice. Season with salt and pepper to taste.

Bring the soup to a boil, then reduce heat to simmer. Cover and cook for about 30-35 mins, or until the rice is tender and the chicken is cooked through.

Taste and adjust seasoning if necessary.

Ladle the soup into bowls, garnish with fresh parsley, and serve hot.

Nutrition (Per Serving): Calories 380 | Fat 8g | Carbs 35g | Protein 42g

32. Vegetable and Lentil Broth with Fresh Herbs

Preparation Time: 15 mins | Cooking Time: 30 mins | Serving Size: 4

Ingredients:

5 oz carrots, diced

5 oz celery, chopped

5 oz potatoes, peeled and cubed

3.5 oz green lentils, rinsed

1 onion, finely chopped

2 cloves garlic, minced

1 bay leaf

1 tsp olive oil

4 cups low-sodium vegetable broth

1 tbsp fresh parsley, chopped

1 tbsp fresh thyme leaves

Salt and pepper to taste

Instructions:

In a large pot, heat olive oil over medium heat. Add chopped onion and garlic, sauté until softened.

Add carrots, celery, and potatoes to the pot. Cook for 5 mins, stirring occasionally.

Pour in the vegetable broth and add the bay leaf. Bring the mixture to a boil.

Once boiling, reduce heat to a simmer and add the rinsed green lentils. Simmer for 20-25 mins or until lentils are tender.

Season the broth with salt and pepper according to your taste.

Remove the bay leaf and discard it. Stir in fresh parsley and thyme leaves just before serving.

Ladle the Vegetable and Lentil Broth into bowls and serve hot.

Nutrition (Per serving): Calories 250 | Fat 2g | Carbs 45g | Protein 12g

33. Butternut Squash and Apple Soup

Preparation Time: 15 mins | Cooking Time: 30 mins | Serving Size: 4

Ingredients:

1.1 lb butternut squash, peeled and diced

10.5 oz apples, peeled, cored, and chopped

7 oz onions, chopped

2 cloves garlic, minced

1 tbsp olive oil

1 tsp ground cinnamon

1/2 tsp ground nutmeg

1/4 tsp ground ginger

4 cups low-sodium vegetable broth

Salt and pepper to taste

Fresh parsley for garnish (optional)

Instructions:

In a large pot, heat olive oil over medium heat. Add chopped onions and minced garlic, sauté until softened.

Add diced butternut squash, chopped apples, ground cinnamon, ground nutmeg, and ground ginger to the pot. Stir well to combine.

Pour in the low-sodium vegetable broth and bring the mixture to a boil. Reduce the heat, cover, and let it simmer for about 25-30 mins or until the squash is tender.

Use an immersion blender to puree the soup until smooth. Alternatively, transfer the mixture to a blender in batches, blending until smooth.

Season with salt and pepper to taste. Adjust the consistency with additional broth if necessary.

Serve the soup hot, garnished with fresh parsley if desired.

Nutrition (Per Serving): Calories 180 | Fat 5g | Carbs 35g | Protein 2g

34. Turkey and Vegetable Quinoa Chowder

Preparation Time: 15 mins | Cooking Time: 30 mins | Serving Size: 4

Ingredients:

8.8 oz lean ground turkey

2/3 cup quinoa, rinsed and drained

1 medium onion, finely chopped

2 carrots, peeled and diced

2 celery stalks, diced

1 red bell pepper, diced

2 cloves garlic, minced

1 tsp dried thyme

1 tsp dried oregano

1 bay leaf

6 cups low-sodium vegetable broth

7 oz green beans, trimmed and chopped

1 zucchini, diced

Salt and pepper to taste

1 cup unsalted chicken broth

1 tbsp olive oil

Instructions:

In a large pot, heat olive oil over medium heat. Add the ground turkey and cook until browned. Break it into smaller pieces as it cooks.

Add the chopped onion, carrots, celery, and red bell pepper to the pot. Sauté until the vegetables are tender, about 5 mins.

Stir in the minced garlic, thyme, oregano, and bay leaf. Cook for an additional 2 mins until the herbs become fragrant.

Pour in the vegetable broth and unsalted chicken broth. Add the rinsed quinoa to the pot. Bring the mixture to a boil, then reduce the heat to low and let it simmer for 15 mins.

Add the green beans and zucchini to the pot. Continue simmering for an additional 10-15 mins or until the quinoa is cooked through and the vegetables are tender.

Season with salt and pepper to taste. Remove the bay leaf before serving.

Nutrition (Per Serving): Calories 380 | Fat 10g | Carbs 45g | Protein 28g

35. Creamy Cauliflower and Leek Soup (Low-Sodium)

Preparation Time: 15 mins | Cooking Time: 25 mins | Serving Size: 4

Ingredients:

1 lb cauliflower, chopped

8.8 oz leeks, sliced (about 1 cup)

1 medium-sized onion, finely diced

2 cloves garlic, minced

1 tbsp olive oil

4 cups low-sodium vegetable broth

8.8 oz potatoes, peeled and diced

1/2 tsp thyme, dried

Salt substitute to taste

Pepper to taste

1 cup low-fat milk

Chopped chives for garnish

Instructions:

In a large pot, heat olive oil over medium heat. Add diced onions and minced garlic, sauté until softened.

Add sliced leeks to the pot and continue sautéing until they are tender, about 3-5 mins.

Stir in cauliflower, potatoes, and dried thyme. Cook for an additional 5 mins, allowing the vegetables to slightly brown.

Pour in the low-sodium vegetable broth, ensuring it covers the vegetables. Season with salt substitute and pepper to taste.

Bring the soup to a boil, then reduce the heat and simmer for 15-20 mins or until the vegetables are tender.

Using an immersion blender, puree the soup until smooth and creamy.

Stir in low-fat milk and heat the soup for an additional 5 mins, ensuring it is heated through.

Adjust seasoning if necessary and serve hot, garnished with chopped chives.

Nutrition (Per serving): Calories 150 | Fat 5g | Carbs 20g | Protein 6g

36. Turkey and Cranberry Wrap with Spinach

Preparation Time: 15 mins | Cooking Time: 10 mins | Serving Size: 2

Ingredients:

7 oz lean turkey breast, thinly sliced

3.5 oz fresh spinach leaves

1.76 oz dried cranberries

2 whole-grain wraps (approx. 1.4 oz each)

2.1 oz low-fat cream cheese

1 oz walnuts, chopped

0.35 oz fresh parsley, chopped

Salt and pepper to taste

Instructions:

Preparation:

Thinly slice the turkey breast.

Wash and dry the fresh spinach leaves.

Chop the walnuts and fresh parsley.

Cooking:

In a non-stick pan over medium heat, cook the turkey slices until fully cooked, approximately 4-5 mins per side. Season with salt and pepper to taste.

Warm the whole-grain wraps in the pan for about 30 seconds on each side.

Assembly:

Spread a layer of low-fat cream cheese on each wrap.

Place the cooked turkey slices on top.

Add a handful of fresh spinach leaves.

Sprinkle dried cranberries, chopped walnuts, and fresh parsley over the ingredients.

Rolling:

Fold in the sides of the wrap and then roll it tightly from the bottom, creating a secure wrap.

Serving:

Slice the wraps in half diagonally for easier handling.

Nutrition (Per Serving): Calories 400 | Fat 15g | Carbs 35g | Protein 30g

37. Grilled Salmon and Avocado Whole Grain Wrap

Preparation Time: 15 mins | Cooking Time: 10 mins | Serving Size: 2 portions

Ingredients:

10.6 oz fresh salmon fillet

4 whole grain wraps (approx. 2.1 oz each)

1 ripe avocado, sliced

1 cup cherry tomatoes, halved

1/2 red onion, thinly sliced

1 tbsp olive oil

1 tsp lemon juice

Salt and pepper to taste

1 tsp dried dill

1/2 tsp garlic powder

Instructions:

Preheat the grill to medium-high heat.

Season the salmon fillet with salt, pepper, dried dill, and garlic powder.

Grill the salmon for about 4-5 mins per side or until it flakes easily with a fork. Remove from the grill and let it rest for a few mins.

In a small bowl, mix olive oil and lemon juice. Drizzle over the sliced avocado to prevent browning.

Warm the whole grain wraps according to the package instructions.

Assemble the wraps by placing a portion of grilled salmon in the center of each wrap.

Top with sliced avocado, cherry tomatoes, and red onion.

Fold the sides of the wrap over the ingredients and roll tightly.

Serve immediately, and enjoy your Grilled Salmon and Avocado Whole Grain Wrap!

Nutrition (Per Serving): Calories 480 | Fat 25g | Carbs 38g | Protein 30g

38. Egg Salad Lettuce Wraps with Fresh Herbs

Preparation Time: 15 mins | Cooking Time: 10 mins | Serving Size: 2

Ingredients:

7 oz hard-boiled eggs, chopped

3.5 oz Greek yogurt (low-fat)

1 oz celery, finely chopped

0.7 oz green onions, thinly sliced

0.35 oz fresh dill, chopped

0.35 oz fresh parsley, chopped

1 tsp Dijon mustard

Salt and pepper to taste

4 large lettuce leaves (Romaine or Bibb)

Instructions:

In a mixing bowl, combine the chopped hard-boiled eggs, Greek yogurt, celery, green onions, fresh dill, fresh parsley, Dijon mustard, salt, and pepper.

Mix the ingredients thoroughly until well combined, ensuring the egg salad has a creamy consistency.

Wash and dry the lettuce leaves, then lay them flat on a clean surface.

Spoon the egg salad mixture onto the center of each lettuce leaf, distributing it evenly.

Carefully fold the sides of the lettuce leaves over the egg salad to create a wrap.

Serve immediately and enjoy the refreshing Egg Salad Lettuce Wraps with Fresh Herbs.

Nutrition (Per Serving): Calories 220 | Fat 12g | Carbs 8g | Protein 18g

39. Mediterranean Hummus and Veggie Sandwich

Preparation Time: 15 mins | Cooking Time: 0 mins | Serving Size: 4

Ingredients:

7 oz canned chickpeas, drained

1.76 oz tahini

1 clove garlic, minced

2 tbsp lemon juice

1 tbsp olive oil

1/2 tsp cumin

Salt and pepper to taste

8 slices whole grain bread

5.3 oz cucumber, thinly sliced

5.3 oz tomatoes, sliced

3.5 oz red bell pepper, thinly sliced

1.76 oz red onion, thinly sliced

1 oz black olives, sliced

Fresh basil leaves for garnish

Instructions:

In a food processor, combine chickpeas, tahini, minced garlic, lemon juice, olive oil, cumin, salt, and pepper. Blend until smooth.

Toast the whole grain bread slices.

Spread a generous layer of the prepared hummus on each slice of toasted bread.

Arrange cucumber slices, tomato slices, red bell pepper slices, red onion slices, and black olives on top of the hummus.

Garnish with fresh basil leaves.

Close the sandwich with another slice of toasted bread.

Nutrition (Per serving): Calories 350 | Fat 15g | Carbs 45g | Protein 10g

40. Chicken and Pesto Caprese Panini with Low-Phosphorus Bread

Preparation Time: 15 mins | Cooking Time: 10 mins | Serving Size: 2 or 4 persons

Ingredients:

7 oz boneless, skinless chicken breast

8 slices of low-phosphorus bread

3.5 oz fresh mozzarella cheese, sliced

1 large tomato, thinly sliced

1 oz fresh basil leaves

2 tbsp pesto sauce (low-phosphorus)

2 tsp unsalted butter (for grilling)

Salt and pepper to taste

Instructions:

Season the chicken breast with salt and pepper. Grill or pan-cook until fully cooked. Allow it to rest for a few mins, then slice it into thin strips.

Lay out the slices of low-phosphorus bread. On one side of each slice, spread a thin layer of low-phosphorus pesto sauce.

Place the sliced chicken evenly on half of the bread slices.

On top of the chicken, add slices of fresh mozzarella, followed by tomato slices and fresh basil leaves.

Place the remaining slices of bread on top, pesto side down, creating sandwiches.

Heat a pan or grill pan over medium heat. Spread a small amount of unsalted butter on the outside of each sandwich.

Grill the sandwiches until the bread is golden brown, and the cheese has melted, approximately 3-5 mins per side.

Once done, remove the panini from the heat, and let them cool for a minute before slicing.

Nutrition (Per serving): Calories 167 | Fat 7 g | Carbs 6 g | Protein 2 g

Dinner

41. Grilled Lemon Herb Salmon with Quinoa

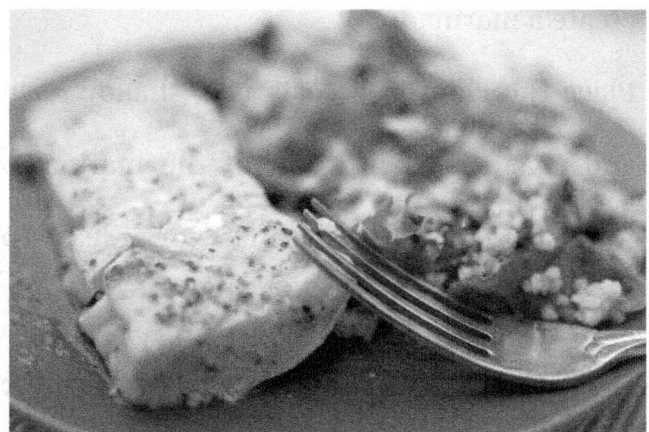

Preparation Time: 15 mins | Cooking Time: 15 mins | Serving Size: 2-4

Ingredients:

14 oz fresh salmon fillets

1 cup quinoa, rinsed

1 lemon, zested and juiced

2 tbsp olive oil

2 cloves garlic, minced

1 tsp dried oregano

1 tsp dried thyme

Salt and pepper to taste

7 oz cherry tomatoes, halved

3.5 oz baby spinach

Instructions:

Prepare the Salmon:

Preheat the grill to medium-high heat.

In a small bowl, mix together half of the lemon zest, half of the lemon juice, 1 tbsp olive oil, minced garlic, oregano, thyme, salt, and pepper.

Place the salmon fillets in a shallow dish and coat them with the lemon herb marinade. Let them marinate for 10 mins.

Cook the Quinoa:

In a medium-sized pot, bring 400ml of water to a boil. Add the rinsed quinoa and reduce heat to low. Cover and simmer for 12-15 mins or until the quinoa is tender and water is absorbed. Fluff with a fork.

Grill the Salmon:

Grill the marinated salmon fillets for about 3-4 mins per side, or until the salmon flakes easily with a fork and has a nice grilled texture.

Prepare the Quinoa Salad:

In a large bowl, combine the cooked quinoa, cherry tomatoes, baby spinach, remaining lemon zest, remaining lemon juice, and 1 tbsp olive oil. Toss until well combined.

Serve:

Divide the quinoa salad among plates and top with grilled lemon herb salmon fillets.

Nutrition (Per serving): Calories 235 | Fat 16 g | Carbs 27 g | Protein 18 g

42. Baked Rosemary Chicken Breast with Steamed Vegetables

Preparation Time: 15 mins | Cooking Time: 25 mins | Serving Size: 2

Ingredients:

14 oz chicken breast, boneless and skinless

1 cup broccoli, florets

2/3 cup carrots, sliced

1/2 cup green beans, trimmed

2 tbsp olive oil

1 tsp dried rosemary

1/2 tsp garlic powder

Salt and pepper to taste

Instructions:

Preheat the oven to 200°C (180°C for fan ovens).

In a small bowl, mix olive oil, dried rosemary, garlic powder, salt, and pepper to create a marinade.

Place the chicken breasts in a shallow dish and coat them with half of the marinade. Allow the chicken to marinate for at least 10 mins.

While the chicken is marinating, prepare the vegetables. Steam broccoli, carrots, and green beans until they are tender yet still crisp. This should take about 5-7 mins.

Heat a non-stick skillet over medium-high heat. Sear the marinated chicken breasts for 2-3 mins on each side or until golden brown.

Transfer the seared chicken breasts to a baking dish and brush them with the remaining marinade.

Bake in the preheated oven for 20-25 mins or until the chicken is cooked through and no longer pink in the center.

In the last 10 mins of baking, place the steamed vegetables around the chicken in the baking dish to finish cooking.

Once done, remove from the oven and let it rest for a few mins before serving.

Nutrition (Per serving): Calories 450 | Fat 18g | Carbs 15g | Protein 55g

43. Garlic Parmesan Crusted Tilapia

Preparation Time: 15 mins | Cooking Time: 15 mins | Serving Size: 2

Ingredients:

21 oz Tilapia fillets

1/3 cup Parmesan cheese, grated

2 tbsp Almond flour

2 cloves Garlic, minced

1 tsp Dried oregano

1 tsp Dried parsley

1/2 tsp Paprika

1/4 tsp Black pepper, freshly ground

1/4 tsp Salt

2 tbsp Olive oil

Lemon wedges for serving

Instructions:

Preheat the oven to 200°C (180°C fan) and line a baking sheet with parchment paper.

In a bowl, combine the grated Parmesan cheese, almond flour, minced garlic, dried oregano, dried parsley, paprika, black pepper, and salt. Mix well.

Pat the tilapia fillets dry with paper towels. Brush each fillet with olive oil.

Dip each tilapia fillet into the Parmesan mixture, pressing the mixture onto the fillets to create an even crust.

Place the coated fillets on the prepared baking sheet.

Bake in the preheated oven for 12-15 mins or until the tilapia is cooked through and the crust is golden brown.

Serve the Garlic Parmesan Crusted Tilapia with lemon wedges.

Nutrition (Per serving): Calories 320 | Fat 18g | Carbs 4g | Protein 35g

44. Lemon Dill Grilled Chicken Skewers

Preparation Time: 15 mins | Cooking Time: 15 mins | Serving Size: 4 persons

Ingredients:

21 oz boneless, skinless chicken breasts, cut into cubes

2 tbsp fresh dill, finely chopped

2 lemons, zest and juice

2 tbsp olive oil

2 cloves garlic, minced

1 tsp dried oregano

Salt and pepper to taste

Wooden skewers, soaked in water for 30 mins

Instructions:

In a bowl, combine the fresh dill, lemon zest, lemon juice, olive oil, minced garlic, dried oregano, salt, and pepper. Mix well to create the marinade.

Place the chicken cubes in a large resealable plastic bag or a shallow dish. Pour the marinade over the chicken, ensuring it's evenly coated. Seal the bag or cover the dish and refrigerate for at least 2 hours, or preferably overnight.

Preheat the grill to medium-high heat.

Thread the marinated chicken cubes onto the soaked wooden skewers.

Grill the chicken skewers for about 6-8 mins per side or until fully cooked and slightly charred. Make sure to turn them occasionally for even cooking.

Once the chicken is cooked through, remove the skewers from the grill.

Serve the Lemon Dill Grilled Chicken Skewers hot, accompanied by your favorite side dishes.

Nutrition (Per Serving): Calories: 189 | Fat: 6 g | Carbs: 9 g | Protein: 10 g

45. Spicy Blackened Cod with Roasted Asparagus

Preparation Time: 15 mins | Cooking Time: 20 mins | Serving Size: 2

Ingredients:

14 oz fresh cod fillets

1 cup asparagus, trimmed

4 tsp olive oil

1 tsp paprika

1/2 tsp garlic powder

1/2 tsp onion powder

1/2 tsp thyme

1/2 tsp oregano

1/2 tsp cayenne pepper (adjust to taste)

Salt and pepper to taste

Instructions:

Preheat the oven to 200°C (392°F).

In a small bowl, mix together paprika, garlic powder, onion powder, thyme, oregano, cayenne pepper, salt, and pepper to create the blackening spice blend.

Pat the cod fillets dry with a paper towel and generously coat each side with the blackening spice blend.

Heat olive oil in an oven-safe skillet over medium-high heat. Once hot, add the cod fillets and sear for 2-3 mins on each side until a blackened crust forms.

Transfer the skillet to the preheated oven and bake for an additional 10-12 mins, or until the cod is cooked through and flakes easily with a fork.

While the cod is baking, toss the trimmed asparagus with olive oil, salt, and pepper. Spread them on a baking sheet and roast in the oven for 10-12 mins or until tender.

Once the cod and asparagus are done, serve them together on a plate.

Nutrition (Per serving): Calories 350 | Fat 15g | Carbs 8g | Protein 45g

46. Pesto Baked Chicken Thighs with Green Beans

Preparation Time: 15 mins | Cooking Time: 30 mins | Serving Size: 4

Ingredients:

1.3 lb chicken thighs, bone-in, skin-on

14 oz fresh green beans, trimmed

2 oz grated Parmesan cheese

2 tbsp pine nuts

2 cloves garlic, minced

1 cup fresh basil leaves

1/2 cup extra-virgin olive oil

Salt and pepper to taste

Instructions:

Preheat the oven to 200°C (180°C fan).

In a food processor, combine Parmesan cheese, pine nuts, minced garlic, and fresh basil leaves. Pulse until finely chopped.

With the processor running, slowly pour in the olive oil until the mixture forms a smooth pesto. Season with salt and pepper to taste.

Place the chicken thighs in a large mixing bowl. Add half of the prepared pesto and toss until the chicken is evenly coated.

Arrange the chicken thighs on one side of a baking sheet lined with parchment paper.

In the same mixing bowl, toss the trimmed green beans with the remaining pesto until well coated.

Place the green beans on the other side of the baking sheet, ensuring they are in a single layer.

Bake in the preheated oven for 25-30 mins or until the chicken is cooked through and the green beans are tender.

Remove from the oven and let it rest for a few mins before serving.

Nutrition (Per serving): Calories: 78 | Fat: 1 g | Carbs: 2 g | Protein: 3 g

47. Teriyaki Glazed Salmon with Brown Rice

Preparation Time: 15 mins | Cooking Time: 20 mins | Serving Size: 4

Ingredients:

1.3 lb fresh salmon fillets

1 cup brown rice (uncooked)

1/4 cup low-sodium soy sauce

2 tbsp mirin

2 tbsp sake

1 tbsp honey (or a sugar substitute for a renal diet)

1 tsp grated ginger

2 cloves garlic, minced

1 tbsp sesame oil

1 tbsp cornstarch (optional, for thickening)

Chopped green onions and sesame seeds for garnish

Instructions:

Prepare Brown Rice:

Rinse 200g of brown rice thoroughly.

Cook the brown rice according to package instructions.

Prepare Salmon:

Preheat the oven to 200°C (180°C fan).

Place salmon fillets on a baking sheet lined with parchment paper.

Season with a pinch of salt and pepper.

Teriyaki Glaze:

In a saucepan, combine soy sauce, mirin, sake, honey (or substitute), grated ginger, and minced garlic.

Cook over medium heat for 5-7 mins, or until the sauce thickens slightly.

Remove from heat and stir in sesame oil.

Optional: Mix cornstarch with a little water and add to the sauce for extra thickness.

Glaze the Salmon:

Brush the teriyaki glaze over the salmon fillets.

Bake:

Bake in the preheated oven for 15-18 mins or until the salmon is cooked through and flakes easily with a fork.

Serve:

Serve the teriyaki glazed salmon over a bed of cooked brown rice.

Drizzle additional teriyaki glaze over the top.

Garnish with chopped green onions and sesame seeds.

Nutrition (Per serving): Calories 350 | Fat 15g | Carbs 25g | Protein 28g

48. Mediterranean Herb Crusted Snapper

Preparation Time: 20 mins | Cooking Time: 15 mins | Serving Size: 4

Ingredients:

14 oz Snapper fillets

1/4 cup fresh parsley, finely chopped

3 tbsp fresh basil, finely chopped

2 tbsp fresh oregano, finely chopped

2 cloves garlic, minced

2 oz whole wheat breadcrumbs

2 oz Parmesan cheese, grated

1 lemon, zest and juice

2 tbsp olive oil

Salt and pepper to taste

Instructions:

Preheat your oven to 200°C (392°F).

In a bowl, combine chopped parsley, basil, oregano, minced garlic, whole wheat breadcrumbs, Parmesan cheese, lemon zest, and olive oil. Mix well to form a herb crust.

Season the snapper fillets with salt and pepper. Place them on a baking sheet lined with parchment paper.

Spread the herb crust evenly over the top of each snapper fillet, pressing it down gently to adhere.

Drizzle lemon juice over the fillets for added flavor.

Bake in the preheated oven for approximately 15 mins or until the crust is golden brown, and the fish is cooked through.

While the snapper is baking, prepare a side salad or steamed vegetables to complement the dish.

Once done, remove from the oven and serve immediately.

Nutrition (Per Serving): Calories 320 | Fat 14g | Carbs 10g | Protein 40g

49. Cilantro Lime Grilled Chicken with Zucchini Noodles

Preparation Time: 20 mins | Cooking Time: 15 mins | Serving Size: 4

Ingredients:

1.3 lb boneless, skinless chicken breasts

1.75 lb zucchini, spiralized into noodles

1/4 cup fresh cilantro, chopped

3 limes, juiced and zested

2 cloves garlic, minced

2 tbsp olive oil

1 tsp ground cumin

Salt and pepper to taste

Instructions:

Marinate the Chicken:

In a bowl, combine lime juice, lime zest, minced garlic, chopped cilantro, olive oil, ground cumin, salt, and pepper.

Place the chicken breasts in a resealable plastic bag and pour half of the marinade over them. Seal the bag and refrigerate for at least 15 mins.

Grill the Chicken:

Preheat the grill to medium-high heat.

Remove the chicken from the marinade and grill for about 6-8 mins per side or until fully cooked.

Brush with the remaining marinade during grilling.

Prepare Zucchini Noodles:

While the chicken is grilling, heat a pan over medium heat.

Add a tbsp of olive oil and sauté the zucchini noodles for 3-4 mins until tender but still crisp.

Assemble the Dish:

Slice the grilled chicken into strips.

Serve the chicken strips on a bed of zucchini noodles.

Nutrition (Per serving): Calories 320 | Fat 12g | Carbs 10g | Protein 40g

50. Baked Herb-Crusted Haddock with Cauliflower Mash

Preparation Time: 15 mins | Cooking Time: 25 mins | Serving Size: 2

Ingredients:

14 oz Haddock fillets

1.1 lb Cauliflower, chopped

2 tbsp Olive oil

1 tsp Dijon mustard

1 tbsp Fresh parsley, chopped

1 tbsp Fresh chives, chopped

1 clove Garlic, minced

1/2 tsp Dried thyme

Salt and pepper to taste

Instructions:

Preheat the oven to 200°C (392°F).

Herb-Crusted Haddock: a. In a small bowl, mix together olive oil, Dijon mustard, minced garlic, chopped parsley, chives, dried thyme, salt, and pepper. b. Place haddock fillets on a baking sheet lined with parchment paper. c. Brush the herb mixture evenly over the haddock fillets, ensuring they are well-coated. d. Bake in the preheated oven for 15-20 mins or until the haddock is cooked through and the crust is golden brown.

Cauliflower Mash: a. While the haddock is baking, steam the chopped cauliflower until tender. b. Place the steamed cauliflower in a food processor and blend until smooth. c. Season the cauliflower mash with salt and pepper to taste.

Serving: a. Divide the cauliflower mash between two plates. b. Place the herb-crusted haddock fillets on top of the cauliflower mash.

Nutrition (Per Serving): Calories 350 | Fat 15g | Carbs 10g | Protein 45g

51. Chickpea and Spinach Curry

Preparation Time: 15 mins | Cooking Time: 25 mins | Serving Size: 4 persons

Ingredients:

14 oz chickpeas, cooked

10.5 oz fresh spinach, washed and chopped

7 oz tomatoes, diced

5.3 oz onions, finely chopped

3.5 oz carrots, diced

2 cloves garlic, minced

1 tbsp ginger, grated

2 tbsp olive oil

1 tsp cumin seeds

1 tsp coriander powder

1 tsp turmeric powder

1 tsp garam masala

1/2 tsp chili powder (adjust to taste)

Salt to taste

Fresh coriander leaves for garnish

Instructions:

In a large pan, heat olive oil over medium heat. Add cumin seeds and let them splutter. Add chopped onions and sauté until golden brown.

Stir in minced garlic and grated ginger, sauté for an additional minute.

Add diced tomatoes, coriander powder, turmeric powder, chili powder, and salt. Cook until the tomatoes are soft and oil begins to separate.

Add diced carrots and cooked chickpeas. Mix well and cook for 5 mins.

Pour in enough water to achieve your desired consistency, then bring the curry to a simmer.

Add chopped spinach and garam masala. Simmer for an additional 5-7 mins until the spinach wilts.

Adjust seasoning according to taste. Garnish with fresh coriander leaves.

Nutrition (Per serving): Calories 320 | Fat 10g | Carbs 45g | Protein 15g

52. Black Bean and Quinoa Stuffed Peppers

Preparation Time: 20 mins | Cooking Time: 40 mins | Serving Size: 4

Ingredients:

1 cup cooked and drained black beans (low sodium or no salt added, rinsed)

3/4 cup quinoa, rinsed

4 large bell peppers, halved and seeds removed

1 tbsp olive oil

1 medium onion, finely chopped

2 cloves garlic, minced

1 tsp ground cumin

1 tsp chili powder (low sodium)

1/2 tsp paprika

1 can (14.5 oz) diced tomatoes, drained (low sodium or no salt added)

1/2 cup corn kernels (fresh or frozen)

Salt (optional) and pepper to taste

Fresh cilantro, chopped (for garnish)

Instructions:

Preheat the Oven: Preheat your oven to 350°F (175°C).

Cook Quinoa: In a medium saucepan, combine the rinsed quinoa with 1.5 cups of water. Bring to a boil, then reduce heat and simmer until quinoa is cooked and water is absorbed (about 15 mins).

Prepare Bell Peppers: While the quinoa is cooking, halve the bell peppers and remove the seeds. Place them in a baking dish.

Sauté Onion and Garlic: In a skillet, heat olive oil over medium heat. Add chopped onion and garlic, sauté until softened.

Add Spices: Stir in cumin, chili powder, and paprika. Cook for an additional minute to release the flavors.

Combine Ingredients: In the skillet, mix the cooked quinoa, black beans, diced tomatoes, and corn. Season with pepper to taste. Cook for another 5 mins until well combined.

Stuff Peppers: Stuff each bell pepper half with the quinoa and black bean mixture, pressing down gently.

Bake: Cover the baking dish with foil and bake in the preheated oven for 25-30 mins, until peppers are tender.

Serve: Remove from the oven and sprinkle chopped cilantro on top. Serve hot.

Nutrition (Per Serving): Calories 350 | Fat 7g | Carbs 60g | Protein 12g

53. Creamy Tuscan White Bean Pasta

Preparation Time: 15 mins | Cooking Time: 20 mins | Serving Size: 4

Ingredients:

12 oz whole grain pasta

1 can (15 oz) white beans, drained and rinsed (low sodium)

1 cup cherry tomatoes, halved

1 1/2 cups fresh spinach, chopped

1 small onion, finely diced

2 cloves garlic, minced

3/4 cup low-sodium vegetable broth

2/3 cup unsweetened almond milk

2 tbsp olive oil

1 tsp dried oregano

1 tsp dried basil

Salt (optional) and pepper to taste

2 tbsp nutritional yeast (optional, for added flavor)

Instructions:

Cook the whole grain pasta according to package instructions. Drain and set aside.

In a large pan, heat olive oil over medium heat. Add diced onion and minced garlic. Sauté until the onion is translucent.

Add cherry tomatoes and cook for 2-3 mins until they begin to soften.

Stir in the white beans, chopped spinach, dried oregano, and dried basil. Cook for an additional 3-4 mins.

Pour in the low-sodium vegetable broth and unsweetened almond milk. Bring the mixture to a simmer.

Add the cooked pasta to the pan, tossing to coat it evenly with the creamy sauce. Cook for an additional 2-3 mins until everything is well combined and heated through.

Season with pepper to taste. If desired, sprinkle nutritional yeast over the pasta for extra flavor.

Serve the Creamy Tuscan White Bean Pasta in individual bowls.

Nutrition (Per Serving): Calories 450 | Fat 10g | Carbs 75g | Protein 20g

54. Sweet Potato and Chickpea Buddha Bowl

Preparation Time: 15 mins | Cooking Time: 30 mins | Serving Size: 2-4 persons

Ingredients:

10.5 oz sweet potatoes, peeled and diced

8.5 oz canned chickpeas, drained and rinsed

3.5 oz quinoa

5.3 oz cherry tomatoes, halved

2.8 oz cucumber, diced

2.1 oz red bell pepper, sliced

1.4 oz red onion, finely chopped

2 tbsp olive oil

1 tsp ground cumin

1 tsp smoked paprika

Salt and pepper to taste

Fresh parsley for garnish

Instructions:

Preheat the oven to 200°C (180°C fan).

Prepare the Sweet Potatoes and Chickpeas:

In a bowl, toss the sweet potatoes and chickpeas with olive oil, ground cumin, smoked paprika, salt, and pepper.

Spread them on a baking sheet in a single layer and roast in the preheated oven for 25-30 mins or until golden and tender, stirring halfway.

Cook the Quinoa:

Rinse the quinoa under cold water.

In a saucepan, combine quinoa with 2 cups of water. Bring to a boil, then reduce heat, cover, and simmer for 15 mins or until the quinoa is cooked and water is absorbed.

Prepare the Dressing:

In a small bowl, whisk together olive oil, lemon juice, minced garlic, Dijon mustard, salt, and pepper.

Assemble the Buddha Bowls:

Divide cooked quinoa among serving bowls.

Top with roasted sweet potatoes and chickpeas, cherry tomatoes, cucumber, red bell pepper, and red onion.

Drizzle the dressing over the bowls.

Garnish and Serve:

Garnish with fresh parsley.

Serve immediately.

Nutrition (Per Serving): Calories 400 | Fat 18g | Carbs 52g | Protein 12g

55. Red Lentil Dal with Coconut Milk

Preparation Time: 15 mins | Cooking Time: 25 mins | Serving Size: 4

Ingredients:

1 cup red lentils

1 large onion, finely chopped

2 cloves garlic, minced

1 tbsp ginger, grated

1 tsp cumin seeds

1 tsp ground coriander

1 tsp turmeric powder

1/2 tsp cinnamon

1/2 tsp cayenne pepper (adjust to taste, optional)

13.5 oz can coconut milk (light, if preferred)

14.5 oz can diced tomatoes (low sodium or no salt added)

1 tbsp vegetable oil

Salt (optional) and pepper to taste

Fresh cilantro for garnish

Instructions:

Rinse the red lentils under cold water until the water runs clear. Set aside.

In a large pot, heat vegetable oil over medium heat. Add cumin seeds and let them sizzle.

Add chopped onions, minced garlic, and grated ginger. Sauté until the onions are soft and golden brown.

Stir in ground coriander, turmeric, cinnamon, and cayenne pepper. Cook for an additional 1-2 mins to release the flavors.

Add the rinsed red lentils and diced tomatoes to the pot. Stir well to combine with the spices.

Pour in the coconut milk and add salt (optional) and pepper to taste. Bring the mixture to a boil.

Reduce heat to low, cover the pot, and let it simmer for about 20 mins or until the lentils are tender.

Once cooked, garnish with fresh cilantro. Adjust salt and spice levels if needed.

Serve the Red Lentil Dal over rice or with your favorite flatbread.

Nutrition (Per Serving): Calories 350 | Fat 15g | Carbs 45g | Protein 15g

56. Mediterranean Three-Bean Salad

Preparation Time: 15 mins | Cooking Time: 0 mins | Serving Size: 4

Ingredients:

5 oz green beans, trimmed and halved

5 oz wax beans, trimmed and halved

1 cup kidney beans, canned, drained, and rinsed

1/2 cup red onion, thinly sliced

1/2 cup cherry tomatoes, halved

1/4 cup Kalamata olives, pitted and sliced

2 tbsp fresh parsley, chopped

For the Dressing:

2 tbsp extra-virgin olive oil

1 tbsp red wine vinegar

1 tsp minced garlic

1 tsp Dijon mustard

Salt and pepper to taste

Instructions:

Prepare the Beans:

Steam the green and wax beans until tender-crisp, about 3-4 mins. Plunge them into cold water to stop the cooking process.

Assemble the Salad:

In a large bowl, combine the steamed beans, kidney beans, red onion, cherry tomatoes, olives, and parsley.

Make the Dressing:

In a small bowl, whisk together the olive oil, red wine vinegar, minced garlic, Dijon mustard, salt, and pepper.

Combine and Toss:

Pour the dressing over the bean mixture and toss until well coated.

Chill and Serve:

Refrigerate the salad for at least 30 mins to allow the flavors to meld.

Serve:

Serve chilled, and if desired, garnish with additional parsley.

Nutrition (Per Serving): Calories 180 | Fat 7g | Carbs 24g | Protein 6g

57. Spicy Black Bean and Corn Quesadillas

Preparation Time: 15 mins | Cooking Time: 15 mins | Serving Size: 4

Ingredients:

14 oz canned black beans, drained and rinsed

7 oz corn kernels, fresh or frozen

5 oz diced tomatoes

3.5 oz diced red bell pepper

2.8 oz diced red onion

2 cloves garlic, minced

1 tsp ground cumin

1 tsp chili powder

1/2 tsp smoked paprika

1/4 tsp cayenne pepper (adjust to taste)

Salt and pepper to taste

8 whole grain tortillas

7 oz shredded reduced-fat cheese (cheddar or Mexican blend)

1 tbsp olive oil

Fresh cilantro for garnish (optional)

Instructions:

In a large bowl, combine black beans, corn, diced tomatoes, red bell pepper, red onion, minced garlic, ground cumin, chili powder, smoked paprika, cayenne pepper, salt, and pepper. Mix well to combine.

Heat olive oil in a skillet over medium heat. Add the bean and vegetable mixture to the skillet and sauté for about 8-10 mins or until the vegetables are tender. Remove from heat.

Place a tortilla on a clean surface and spoon a portion of the bean and vegetable mixture onto one half of the tortilla. Sprinkle with shredded cheese and fold the other half over to create a quesadilla.

Heat a non-stick pan over medium heat. Cook each quesadilla for 2-3 mins on each side or until the tortilla is golden brown and the cheese is melted.

Repeat the process for the remaining tortillas and filling.

Once cooked, let the quesadillas rest for a minute before slicing them into wedges.

Serve the Spicy Black Bean and Corn Quesadillas warm, garnished with fresh cilantro if desired.

Nutrition (Per Serving): Calories 350 | Fat 10g | Carbs 52g | Protein 15g

58. Quinoa and Black-Eyed Pea Salad

Preparation Time: 15 mins | Cooking Time: 20 mins | Serving Size: 4

Ingredients:

5.3 oz quinoa

7 oz black-eyed peas, cooked and drained

1 cup cucumber, diced

1 cup red bell pepper, diced

1/2 cup red onion, finely chopped

1.8 oz fresh parsley, chopped

1 oz feta cheese, crumbled (optional)

For the Dressing:

3 tbsp olive oil

2 tbsp lemon juice

1 tsp Dijon mustard

1 tsp minced garlic

Salt and pepper to taste

Instructions:

Rinse the quinoa under cold water. In a medium-sized pot, combine the quinoa with 300ml of water. Bring to a boil, then reduce heat, cover, and simmer for 15 mins or until the quinoa is cooked and water is absorbed. Remove from heat and let it cool.

In a large mixing bowl, combine the cooked quinoa, black-eyed peas, cucumber, red bell pepper, red onion, and parsley.

In a small bowl, whisk together the olive oil, lemon juice, Dijon mustard, minced garlic, salt, and pepper to create the dressing.

Pour the dressing over the salad and toss until all ingredients are well coated.

If using, sprinkle crumbled feta cheese over the salad and gently toss again.

Adjust salt and pepper according to taste.

Chill the salad in the refrigerator for at least 1 hour before serving to enhance the flavors.

Nutrition (Per Serving): Calories 320 | Fat 12g | Carbs 42g | Protein 10g

59. Eggplant and Lentil Moussaka

Preparation Time: 30 mins | Cooking Time: 45 mins | Serving Size: 4

Ingredients:

17.6 oz eggplant, thinly sliced

8.8 oz lentils, cooked

14 oz canned tomatoes, crushed

1 cup onion, finely chopped

3 cloves garlic, minced

5.3 oz low-fat feta cheese, crumbled

1.8 oz whole wheat flour

2 cups low-sodium vegetable broth

2 tbsp olive oil

1 tsp dried oregano

1 tsp dried thyme

Salt and pepper to taste

Instructions:

Preheat the oven to 180°C (350°F).

In a large pan, heat 1 tbsp of olive oil over medium heat. Sauté the chopped onion and minced garlic until softened.

Add the sliced eggplant and cook until golden brown. Set aside.

In the same pan, add the whole wheat flour and cook for 2 mins, stirring continuously to avoid lumps.

Gradually whisk in the low-sodium vegetable broth until a smooth sauce forms.

Stir in the crushed tomatoes, cooked lentils, dried oregano, dried thyme, salt, and pepper. Simmer for 10 mins until the sauce thickens.

In a baking dish, layer half of the eggplant slices, followed by half of the lentil-tomato mixture. Repeat with the remaining eggplant and lentil-tomato mixture.

Crumble the low-fat feta cheese evenly over the top layer.

Bake in the preheated oven for 30 mins or until the top is golden and bubbly.

Allow the moussaka to cool for a few mins before serving.

Nutrition (Per Serving): Calories 380 | Fat 12g | Carbs 45g | Protein 20g

60. Lentil and Vegetable Stew

Preparation Time: 15 mins | Cooking Time: 30 mins | Serving Size: 4

Ingredients:

7 oz green lentils, rinsed and drained

1 large onion, finely chopped

2 carrots, diced (5.3 oz)

2 celery stalks, sliced (3.5 oz)

1 red bell pepper, diced (5.3 oz)

2 cloves garlic, minced

14 oz canned diced tomatoes

4 cups low-sodium vegetable broth

1 tsp dried thyme

1 tsp ground cumin

1 bay leaf

Salt and pepper to taste

1 tbsp olive oil

Instructions:

Prepare Lentils:

Rinse the green lentils under cold water and drain.

Sauté Aromatics:

In a large pot, heat olive oil over medium heat.

Add chopped onions and garlic, sauté until softened.

Add Vegetables:

Stir in carrots, celery, and red bell pepper. Sauté for an additional 5 mins.

Seasoning:

Add dried thyme, ground cumin, bay leaf, salt, and pepper. Mix well.

Cook Lentils:

Incorporate the rinsed lentils into the pot and stir to combine.

Pour Broth and Tomatoes:

Pour in the vegetable broth and canned diced tomatoes with their juices. Bring to a simmer.

Simmer:

Reduce heat to low, cover, and let it simmer for about 25-30 mins or until lentils are tender.

Adjust Seasoning:

Taste and adjust salt and pepper according to your preference.

Serve:

Discard the bay leaf before serving.

Nutrition (Per Serving): Calories 320 | Fat 5g | Carbs 55g | Protein 18g

61. Chicken and Mushroom Risotto with Asparagus

Preparation Time: 15 mins | Cooking Time: 30 mins | Serving Size: 4

Ingredients:

10.5 oz chicken breast, diced

1 cup Arborio rice

5.3 oz mushrooms, sliced

7 oz asparagus, trimmed and cut into 2-inch pieces

1 onion, finely chopped

2 cloves garlic, minced

4 cups low-sodium chicken broth

2/3 cup dry white wine

1.8 oz Parmesan cheese, grated

2 tbsp olive oil

Salt and pepper to taste

Fresh parsley, chopped (for garnish)

Instructions:

In a large skillet, heat 1 tbsp of olive oil over medium heat. Add the diced chicken and cook until browned and cooked through. Remove the chicken from the skillet and set aside.

In the same skillet, add another tbsp of olive oil. Sauté the chopped onion and minced garlic until softened.

Add the Arborio rice to the skillet and cook, stirring, for 2-3 mins until the rice is lightly toasted.

Pour in the white wine and cook until it's mostly evaporated, stirring constantly.

Begin adding the chicken broth, one ladle at a time, allowing the liquid to be absorbed before adding more. Continue this process until the rice is creamy and cooked to al dente texture.

In the last 5 mins of cooking, stir in the sliced mushrooms and asparagus pieces. Add salt and pepper to taste.

Once the risotto is cooked, stir in the cooked chicken and grated Parmesan cheese. Adjust seasoning if needed.

Serve the risotto hot, garnished with fresh chopped parsley.

Nutrition (Per Serving): Calories 450 | Fat 12g | Carbs 55g | Protein 30g

62. Mediterranean Vegetable and Rice Casserole

Preparation Time: 20 mins | Cooking Time: 45 mins | Serving Size: 4

Ingredients:

1 cup brown rice

14 oz zucchini, diced

10.5 oz cherry tomatoes, halved

7 oz red bell pepper, chopped

5.3 oz eggplant, cubed

3.5 oz red onion, finely sliced

2 cloves garlic, minced

4 tbsp olive oil

1 tsp dried oregano

1 tsp dried thyme

Salt and pepper to taste

2 cups vegetable broth

Instructions:

Preheat Oven:

Preheat the oven to 180°C (350°F).

Prepare Rice:

Cook the brown rice according to package instructions.

Sauté Vegetables:

In a large pan, heat olive oil over medium heat. Add garlic and onion, sauté until softened.

Add zucchini, cherry tomatoes, red bell pepper, and eggplant. Cook until vegetables are slightly tender.

Season:

Season the vegetables with dried oregano, dried thyme, salt, and pepper. Mix well.

Combine with Rice:

In a large mixing bowl, combine the cooked rice with the sautéed vegetables. Mix thoroughly.

Transfer to Casserole Dish:

Transfer the vegetable and rice mixture to a greased casserole dish.

Add Vegetable Broth:

Pour vegetable broth over the mixture to keep it moist during baking.

Bake:

Cover the casserole dish with foil and bake in the preheated oven for 30 mins. Then, uncover and bake for an additional 15 mins or until the top is golden.

Serve:

Allow the casserole to cool slightly before serving.

Nutrition (Per serving): Calories 350 | Fat 12g | Carbs 52g | Protein 8g

63. Quinoa and Spinach Stuffed Bell Peppers

Preparation Time: 20 mins | Cooking Time: 30 mins | Serving Size: 4 persons

Ingredients:

1 cup quinoa

4 large bell peppers, halved and seeds removed

7 oz fresh spinach, chopped

1 cup cherry tomatoes, diced

1 small red onion, finely chopped

2 cloves garlic, minced

4 oz low-sodium feta cheese, crumbled

1 tsp dried oregano

1 tsp dried thyme

Salt (optional) and pepper to taste

2 tbsp olive oil

Instructions:

Preheat the oven to 350°F (175°C).

Rinse the quinoa under cold water. Cook according to package instructions, substituting water with low-sodium vegetable broth for added flavor.

In a pan, heat olive oil over medium heat. Sauté onion and garlic until softened.

Add spinach to the pan and cook until wilted. Mix in the diced tomatoes and cook for 2 mins.

In a large bowl, combine cooked quinoa, sautéed vegetables, feta cheese, oregano, thyme, and pepper. Adjust seasoning to taste.

Fill each bell pepper half with the quinoa mixture.

Place stuffed peppers in a baking dish, cover with foil, and bake for 20 mins. Remove foil and bake for an additional 10 mins.

Serve warm.

Nutrition (Per serving): Calories 350 | Fat 12g | Carbs 50g | Protein 15g

64. Lemon Herb Baked Cod with Couscous

Preparation Time: 15 mins | Cooking Time: 20 mins | Serving Size: 4

Ingredients:

4 cod fillets (approximately 1.3 lb)

1 cup whole wheat couscous

1 lemon, thinly sliced

2 tbsp olive oil

2 cloves garlic, minced

1 tsp dried oregano

1 tsp dried thyme

1 tsp paprika

Salt (optional) and pepper to taste

Fresh parsley, for garnish

Instructions:

Preheat the oven to 400°F (200°C).

Rinse cod fillets and pat dry. Arrange in a baking dish.

In a bowl, combine olive oil, garlic, oregano, thyme, paprika, and pepper. Brush mixture over cod. Top with lemon slices.

Bake for 15-20 mins, until cod flakes easily.

Prepare couscous according to package instructions, using low-sodium broth.

Serve cod over couscous, garnished with parsley.

Nutrition (Per serving): Calories 350 | Fat 8g | Carbs 30g | Protein 40g

65. Cheesy Broccoli and Chicken Casserole

Preparation Time: 15 mins | Cooking Time: 30 mins | Serving Size: 4 persons

Ingredients:

1.1 lb chicken breasts, diced

14 oz broccoli, cut into florets

7 oz low-fat, low-sodium mozzarella cheese, shredded

5 oz low-fat cheddar cheese, shredded

1 cup low-sodium chicken broth

1 cup low-fat sour cream

2/3 cup low-fat mayonnaise

1 tsp garlic powder

1 tsp onion powder

Salt (optional) and pepper to taste

Cooking spray

Instructions:

Preheat the oven to 375°F (190°C).

Cook chicken in a skillet. Season with garlic powder, onion powder, and pepper.

Steam broccoli until crisp-tender, about 3-4 mins.

In a bowl, mix sour cream, mayonnaise, and chicken broth.

Combine chicken, broccoli, and cheeses in a large bowl.

Grease a casserole dish with cooking spray. Add chicken mixture, pour over the sour cream mixture.

Bake for 25-30 mins until bubbly and golden.

Let cool before serving.

Nutrition (Per serving): Calories 450 | Fat 22g | Carbs 12g | Protein 50g

66. Creamy Tomato Basil Risotto with Grilled Chicken

Preparation Time: 30 mins | Cooking Time: 30 mins | Serving Size: 4 persons

Ingredients:

1.5 cups Arborio rice

4 chicken breasts, grilled and sliced

1 onion, finely chopped

2 cloves garlic, minced

28 oz canned diced tomatoes, low sodium

5 cups low-sodium chicken broth, kept warm

1 cup cherry tomatoes, halved

1 cup fresh basil leaves, chopped

5 oz Parmesan cheese, grated

4 tbsp unsalted butter

Salt (optional) and pepper to taste

Instructions:

In a skillet, melt half the butter over medium heat. Sauté onion and garlic.

Add rice, cook until lightly toasted. Stir in diced tomatoes.

Gradually add chicken broth, stirring until absorbed. Continue until rice is al dente.

Mix in chicken, cherry tomatoes, basil, Parmesan, remaining butter, and season. Serve warm.

Nutrition (Per serving): Calories 480 | Fat 14g | Carbs 58g | Protein 32g

67. Spinach and Feta Stuffed Portobello Mushrooms

Preparation Time: 15 mins | Cooking Time: 25 mins | Serving Size: 4

Ingredients:

4 large Portobello mushrooms

7 oz fresh spinach, chopped

5 oz low-sodium feta cheese, crumbled

1 small onion, finely diced

2 cloves garlic, minced

2 tbsp pine nuts, toasted

2 tbsp olive oil

1 tsp dried oregano

Salt (optional) and pepper to taste

Instructions:

Preheat oven to 400°F (200°C).

Prepare mushrooms, remove stems. Brush caps with olive oil.

Sauté onion and garlic. Add spinach until wilted. Season with oregano and pepper.

Mix spinach with feta and pine nuts. Stuff mushrooms.

Bake for 20-25 mins until tender.

Serve warm

Nutrition (Per Serving): Calories: 123 | Fat: 6 g | Carbs: 9 g | Protein: 5 g

68. Mexican Quinoa Casserole with Black Beans

Preparation Time: 15 mins | Cooking Time: 30 mins | Serving Size: 4

Ingredients:

7 oz quinoa

14 oz black beans, cooked and drained

7 oz corn kernels

1 red bell pepper, diced

1 yellow bell pepper, diced

1 onion, finely chopped

2 cloves garlic, minced

1 tsp ground cumin

1 tsp chili powder

1 tsp smoked paprika

14 oz diced tomatoes, canned

5.3 oz shredded cheddar cheese

Fresh cilantro, chopped (for garnish)

Salt and pepper to taste

Olive oil for cooking

Instructions:

Preparation:

Rinse quinoa under cold water.

Cook quinoa according to package instructions.

Preheat the oven to 180°C (350°F).

Cooking:

In a large skillet, heat olive oil over medium heat.

Sauté onions until translucent, then add garlic and cook until fragrant.

Add diced bell peppers and cook until softened.

Stir in ground cumin, chili powder, and smoked paprika.

Pour in diced tomatoes and let the mixture simmer for 5 mins.

Add cooked quinoa, black beans, and corn to the skillet. Mix well.

Season with salt and pepper to taste.

Transfer the mixture to a greased casserole dish and top with shredded cheddar cheese.

Bake in the preheated oven for 20 mins or until the cheese is melted and bubbly.

Serving:

Remove from the oven and let it cool slightly before serving.

Garnish with fresh cilantro.

Nutrition (Per serving): Calories 450 | Fat 12g | Carbs 70g | Protein 18g

69. Lemon Garlic Shrimp and Rice Skillet

Preparation Time: 15 mins | Cooking Time: 20 mins | Serving Size: 4

Ingredients:

14 oz shrimp, peeled and deveined

7 oz long-grain white rice

1 tbsp olive oil

1 onion, finely chopped

3 cloves garlic, minced

1 red bell pepper, diced

1 yellow bell pepper, diced

1 cup cherry tomatoes, halved

1 tsp dried oregano

1 tsp paprika

Salt and black pepper to taste

1/2 cup chicken broth

Zest of 1 lemon

Juice of 1 lemon

Fresh parsley, chopped, for garnish

Instructions:

In a medium-sized pot, cook the rice according to package instructions. Set aside.

In a large skillet, heat olive oil over medium heat. Add chopped onions and minced garlic, sauté until softened.

Add the shrimp to the skillet and cook until they turn pink, about 2-3 mins per side. Remove shrimp from the skillet and set aside.

In the same skillet, add diced bell peppers, halved cherry tomatoes, oregano, paprika, salt, and black pepper. Sauté until the vegetables are tender.

Pour in chicken broth, lemon zest, and lemon juice. Stir well.

Return the cooked shrimp to the skillet and cook for an additional 2-3 mins, allowing the flavors to meld.

Add the cooked rice to the skillet and toss everything together until well combined.

Garnish with fresh chopped parsley before serving.

Nutrition (Per serving): Calories 380 | Fat 8g | Carbs 45g | Protein 30g

70. Sweet Potato and Kale Frittata

Preparation Time: 15 mins | Cooking Time: 25 mins | Serving Size: 4

Ingredients:

14 oz sweet potatoes, peeled and diced

5.3 oz kale, stems removed and chopped

8 large eggs

3.5 oz feta cheese, crumbled

1 small onion, finely chopped

2 cloves garlic, minced

1 tbsp olive oil

1 tsp dried thyme

Salt and pepper to taste

Instructions:

Preheat the Oven:

Preheat your oven to 180°C (350°F).

Steam Sweet Potatoes:

Place the diced sweet potatoes in a steamer basket and steam for 8-10 mins until they are just tender. Set aside.

Sauté Onions and Garlic:

In an oven-safe skillet, heat olive oil over medium heat. Add chopped onions and garlic, sauté until softened.

Add Kale:

Add chopped kale to the skillet and cook until wilted.

Whisk Eggs:

In a bowl, whisk the eggs together. Season with salt, pepper, and dried thyme.

Combine Ingredients:

Add steamed sweet potatoes to the skillet, distributing them evenly. Pour the whisked eggs over the vegetables. Sprinkle crumbled feta cheese on top.

Cook on Stovetop:

Cook on the stovetop over medium heat for 3-4 mins, allowing the edges to set.

Bake:

Transfer the skillet to the preheated oven and bake for 15-18 mins or until the frittata is set in the center.

Serve:

Once cooked, let it cool slightly before slicing. Serve warm.

Nutrition (Per serving): Calories 320 | Fat 18g | Carbs 24g | Protein 15g

Snacks and Teatime

71. Savory Chickpea Delight

Preparation Time: 15 mins | Cooking Time: 25 mins | Serving Size: 4

Ingredients:

14 oz canned chickpeas, drained and rinsed

7 oz cherry tomatoes, halved

5.3 oz cucumber, diced

3.5 oz red bell pepper, chopped

1.8 oz red onion, finely chopped

2 cloves garlic, minced

1 oz fresh parsley, chopped

2 tbsp olive oil

1 tbsp balsamic vinegar

1 tsp ground cumin

1 tsp paprika

Salt and pepper to taste

7 oz feta cheese, crumbled (optional)

Instructions:

In a large mixing bowl, combine the chickpeas, cherry tomatoes, cucumber, red bell pepper, red onion, garlic, and fresh parsley.

In a small bowl, whisk together the olive oil, balsamic vinegar, ground cumin, paprika, salt, and pepper.

Pour the dressing over the chickpea mixture and toss until well combined.

Allow the mixture to marinate for at least 10 mins to let the flavors meld.

If using feta cheese, sprinkle it over the salad just before serving.

Serve the Savory Chickpea Delight in portions, and enjoy!

Nutrition (Per Serving): Calories 320 | Fat 14g | Carbs 38g | Protein 12g

72. Crispy Kale Chips

Preparation Time: 15 mins | Cooking Time: 15 mins | Serving Size: 4

Ingredients:

7 oz fresh kale, washed and thoroughly dried

2 tsp olive oil

1/2 tsp salt (adjust to taste)

1/2 tsp garlic powder

1/2 tsp nutritional yeast (optional)

Instructions:

Preheat your oven to 150°C (300°F).

Remove the tough stems from the kale leaves and tear them into bite-sized pieces.

In a large bowl, combine the kale with olive oil. Massage the oil into the leaves, ensuring they are evenly coated.

Sprinkle salt, garlic powder, and nutritional yeast over the kale, tossing gently to distribute the seasonings evenly.

Line a baking sheet with parchment paper and spread the kale in a single layer, ensuring they are not crowded.

Bake in the preheated oven for 12-15 mins or until the edges are crispy but not burnt, tossing the kale halfway through the cooking time.

Remove from the oven and let the kale chips cool on the baking sheet for a few mins to crisp up further.

Serve immediately and enjoy your crunchy and flavorful Crispy Kale Chips!

Nutrition (Per Serving): Calories 85 | Fat 5g | Carbs 10g | Protein 4g

73. Zesty Guacamole Bruschetta

Preparation Time: 15 mins | Cooking Time: 5 mins | Serving Size: 4

Ingredients:

7 oz ripe avocados, peeled, pitted, and diced

3.5 oz tomatoes, diced

1.75 oz red onion, finely chopped

1 clove garlic, minced

2 tsp fresh cilantro, chopped

1 tbsp lime juice

1 tbsp olive oil

Salt and pepper to taste

4 slices whole grain bread (7 oz)

Instructions:

In a bowl, combine diced avocados, tomatoes, red onion, garlic, and cilantro.

Add lime juice and olive oil to the mixture. Season with salt and pepper according to taste.

Gently toss the ingredients until well combined. Set aside.

Toast the whole grain bread slices until they are golden brown and crispy.

Spoon the zesty guacamole mixture onto each toasted bread slice, spreading it evenly. Serve immediately, and enjoy the vibrant flavors of Zesty Guacamole Bruschetta.

Nutrition (Per Serving): Calories 220 | Fat 15g | Carbs 20g | Protein 4g

74. Spicy Roasted Edamame

Preparation Time: 10 mins | Cooking Time: 20 mins | Serving Size: 4

Ingredients:

14 oz frozen edamame, shelled

2 tbsp olive oil

1 tsp garlic powder

1 tsp onion powder

1 tsp smoked paprika

1/2 tsp cayenne pepper (adjust to taste, optional for renal diet)

1/2 tsp black pepper

1/2 tsp sea salt (use less or omit for renal diet)

1 tbsp low-sodium soy sauce

1 tsp sesame oil

Instructions:

Preheat your oven to 400°F (200°C).

Thaw and shell the edamame if not pre-shelled.

In a mixing bowl, toss the edamame with olive oil, garlic powder, onion powder, smoked paprika, cayenne pepper (if using), black pepper, and sea salt.

Spread the edamame on a baking sheet in a single layer.

Roast in the oven for 15-20 mins or until golden and slightly crispy, stirring halfway through.

Mix soy sauce and sesame oil in a small bowl, drizzle over the roasted edamame, and toss to coat.

Let cool slightly before serving.

Nutrition (Per Serving): Calories: 234 | Fat: 12 g | Carbs: 16 g | Protein: 16 g

75. Tomato Basil Quinoa Bites

Preparation Time: 20 mins | Cooking Time: 25 mins | Serving Size: 4

Ingredients:

1 cup quinoa, rinsed

1 3/4 cups low-sodium vegetable broth

2 large eggs

1/2 cup grated Parmesan cheese

1 cup cherry tomatoes, diced

1/4 cup fresh basil, finely chopped

2 cloves garlic, minced

1/2 tsp salt (adjust to taste, or omit for renal diet)

1/4 tsp black pepper

Cooking spray

Instructions:

Preheat the oven to 375°F (190°C). Cook quinoa in low-sodium vegetable broth until fluffy and liquid is absorbed. Let cool.

In a large bowl, mix cooled quinoa, eggs, Parmesan, tomatoes, basil, garlic, salt (if using), and pepper.

Grease a mini muffin tin with cooking spray. Spoon the quinoa mixture into the tin, pressing down lightly.

Bake for 20-25 mins or until the edges are golden.

Let cool before serving.

Nutrition (Per serving): Calories 220 | Fat 7g | Carbs 30g | Protein 10g

76. Tropical Paradise Parfait

Preparation Time: 15 mins | Cooking Time: 0 mins | Serving Size: 2

Ingredients:

7 oz fresh pineapple, diced

5.3 oz mango, peeled and diced

3.5 oz papaya, diced

7 oz low-fat Greek yogurt (low sodium)

2 tbsp unsweetened shredded coconut

2 tbsp slivered almonds

2 tsp chia seeds

1 tbsp honey (optional, or use a suitable sugar substitute)

Instructions:

Mix pineapple, mango, and papaya in a bowl.

Stir chia seeds into Greek yogurt and let sit for 5 mins.

Layer yogurt-chia mixture and fruit in serving glasses, starting with yogurt.

Sprinkle each layer with coconut and almonds.

Drizzle with honey if desired and garnish with mint leaves.

Serve immediately

Nutrition (Per serving): Calories 320 | Fat 12g | Carbs 45g | Protein 12g

77. Berries and Cream Delight

Preparation Time: 15 mins | Cooking Time: 0 mins | Serving Size: 4

Ingredients:

17.5 oz mixed berries (strawberries, blueberries, raspberries)

7 oz low-fat Greek yogurt

3.5 oz low-fat whipped cream

1 oz powdered erythritol (or preferred sugar substitute)

1 tsp vanilla extract

2 tsp chia seeds

Fresh mint leaves for garnish

Instructions:

Prepare the Berries:

Wash and hull the strawberries.

In a mixing bowl, combine all the berries.

Make the Cream Mixture:

In a separate bowl, mix the Greek yogurt, whipped cream, powdered erythritol, and vanilla extract.

Stir until well combined.

Assemble the Berries and Cream Delight:

Divide the mixed berries equally into serving bowls.

Layer with Cream Mixture:

Spoon the cream mixture over the berries in each bowl.

Add Chia Seeds:

Sprinkle chia seeds evenly over the cream layer.

Garnish and Chill:

Garnish with fresh mint leaves.

Refrigerate for at least 1 hour to let the flavors meld.

Serve:

Serve chilled and enjoy this delightful, kidney-friendly dessert!

Nutrition (Per Serving): Calories: 156 | Fat: 5 g | Carbs: 2 g | Protein: 4 g

78. Mango Tango Smoothie Bowl

Preparation Time: 10 mins | Cooking Time: 0 mins | Serving Size: 2

Ingredients:

10.5 oz frozen mango chunks

5.25 oz plain low-fat yogurt

1 medium banana, sliced

1 oz chia seeds

0.5 oz honey (optional, based on dietary restrictions)

0.7 oz unsweetened coconut flakes

2 tsp flaxseeds

5 oz unsweetened almond milk

Fresh mint leaves for garnish

Instructions:

In a blender, combine the frozen mango chunks, plain low-fat yogurt, sliced banana, chia seeds, honey (if using), flaxseeds, and unsweetened almond milk.

Blend the ingredients until you achieve a smooth and creamy consistency.

Pour the smoothie mixture into bowls.

Top each bowl with unsweetened coconut flakes and garnish with fresh mint leaves.

Serve immediately and enjoy your refreshing Mango Tango Smoothie Bowl!

Nutrition (Per serving): Calories 320 | Fat 12g | Carbs 50g | Protein 8g

79. Pineapple Coconut Yogurt Popsicles

Preparation Time: 15 mins | Cooking Time: 0 mins | Serving Size: 4

Ingredients:

14 oz fresh pineapple, peeled and diced

7 oz coconut yogurt (low potassium if possible)

2 tbsp honey (or a suitable sugar substitute)

2 tbsp unsweetened shredded coconut

Instructions:

Blend pineapple and coconut yogurt until smooth.

Stir in honey (or substitute) and shredded coconut.

Pour mixture into popsicle molds and insert sticks.

Freeze for at least 4-6 hours or overnight.

To release popsicles, run molds under warm water briefly.

Enjoy your refreshing pineapple coconut yogurt popsicles!

Nutrition (Per serving): Calories 120 | Fat 5g | Carbs 18g | Protein 2g

80. Citrus Burst Fruit Salad

Preparation Time: 15 mins | Cooking Time: 0 mins | Serving Size: 4

Ingredients:

8.75 oz strawberries, hulled and sliced

7 oz pineapple, diced

2 oranges, peeled and segmented

1 grapefruit, peeled and segmented

1 kiwi, peeled and sliced

1 banana, sliced

1 oz fresh mint leaves, chopped

Dressing:

1 oz honey

1 tbsp fresh lime juice

1 tsp orange zest

Instructions:

In a large mixing bowl, combine the strawberries, pineapple, oranges, grapefruit, kiwi, banana, and mint leaves.

In a separate small bowl, whisk together the honey, fresh lime juice, and orange zest to create the dressing.

Pour the dressing over the fruit mixture and gently toss until all the fruits are well coated.

Refrigerate the fruit salad for at least 30 mins to allow the flavors to meld.

Serve chilled and garnish with additional mint leaves if desired.

Nutrition (Per Serving): Calories 150 | Fat 0.5g | Carbs 38g | Protein 2g

81. Nutty Banana Oat Bars

Preparation Time: 15 mins | Cooking Time: 25 mins | Serving Size: 4

Ingredients:

7 oz ripe bananas, mashed (about 2 medium bananas)

1 cup rolled oats

1/2 cup chopped nuts (almonds or walnuts)

1/4 cup almond flour

2 tbsp honey or maple syrup (use a suitable sugar substitute for a renal diet)

1 tbsp coconut oil, melted

1 tsp vanilla extract

1/2 tsp ground cinnamon

A pinch of salt

Instructions:

Preheat your oven to 350°F (180°C). Line an 8x8 inch baking pan with parchment paper.

In a large bowl, mix mashed bananas, oats, nuts, almond flour, sweetener, coconut oil, vanilla extract, cinnamon, and salt until well combined.

Press the mixture firmly into the prepared pan.

Bake for 25 mins or until edges are golden brown.

Let cool before cutting into bars.

Nutrition (Per serving): Calories 150 | Fat 8g | Carbs 18g | Protein 4g

1/2 cup rolled oats

2 tbsp chia seeds

2 tbsp almond butter

1 tbsp honey (or use a suitable sugar substitute)

1 tsp vanilla extract

A pinch of salt

Instructions:

Pulse cranberries, almonds, oats, and chia seeds in a food processor until finely chopped.

Add almond butter, sweetener, vanilla, and salt. Pulse until a sticky dough forms.

Roll into 12 bite-sized balls. Chill for 30 mins before serving.

Nutrition (Per Serving): Calories 120 | Fat 6g | Carbs 15g | Protein 3g

82. Cranberry Almond Energy Bites

Preparation Time: 15 mins | Cooking Time: 0 mins | Serving Size: 12 bites

Ingredients:

1 cup dried cranberries

1 cup almonds

83. Date and Walnut Bliss Balls

Preparation Time: 15 mins | Cooking Time: 0 mins | Serving Size: 12 balls

Ingredients:

7 oz pitted dates

1 cup walnuts

2 tbsp chia seeds

2 tbsp unsweetened shredded coconut

1 tsp vanilla extract

1/2 tsp ground cinnamon

A pinch of salt

Instructions:

Process all ingredients in a food processor until a sticky dough forms.

Roll into 12 balls and chill for 30 mins.

Nutrition (Per Serving): Calories: 156 | Fat: 7 g | Carbs: 3 g | Protein: 2 g

84. Chia Seed Pudding Parfait

Preparation Time: 10 mins | Cooking Time: 0 mins | Serving Size: 2-4

Ingredients:

1/4 cup chia seeds

1 cup unsweetened almond milk

1 tbsp honey (optional, adjust based on dietary needs)

1 tsp vanilla extract

1 cup fresh berries

1/4 cup low-fat Greek yogurt

1/4 cup granola (low sodium)

Instructions:

Mix chia seeds, almond milk, sweetener, and vanilla. Chill until pudding consistency.

Layer pudding, berries, yogurt, and granola in serving glasses.

Nutrition (Per Serving): Calories 250 | Fat 10g | Carbs 30g | Protein 8g

85. Blueberry Quinoa Bars

Preparation Time: 15 mins | Cooking Time: 25 mins | Serving Size: 4

Ingredients:

1 cup cooked quinoa

1/2 cup almond flour

1/4 cup coconut flour

1/4 tsp salt

1/2 tsp baking powder

1/4 cup coconut oil, melted

1/4 cup honey (use a sugar substitute if needed)

1 tsp vanilla extract

2 large eggs

1 cup fresh blueberries

Instructions:

Combine quinoa, flours, salt, and baking powder. Add wet ingredients and blueberries. Bake in a lined dish at 350°F for 25 mins.

Nutrition (Per serving): Calories 300 | Fat 15g | Carbs 35g | Protein 8g

Desserts and Sweets

86. Guilt-Free Chocolate Avocado Mousse

Preparation Time: 15 mins | Cooking Time: 0 mins | Serving Size: 2-4

Ingredients:

Ingredients:

2 ripe avocados

1/2 cup unsweetened cocoa powder

1/3 cup powdered erythritol (or suitable sugar substitute)

1/2 cup unsweetened almond milk

1 tsp vanilla extract

A pinch of salt

Optional toppings: chopped nuts, berries

Instructions:

Blend avocados, cocoa powder, sweetener, almond milk, vanilla, and salt until smooth.

Chill for 1 hour before serving with optional toppings.

Nutrition (Per Serving): Calories 180 | Fat 15g | Carbs 10g | Protein 3g

87. Stevia-Sweetened Berry Parfait

Preparation Time: 15 mins | Cooking Time: 0 mins | Serving Size: 2

Ingredients:

5.3 oz fresh strawberries, hulled and sliced

3.5 oz fresh blueberries

3.5 oz fresh raspberries

8.8 oz plain Greek yogurt (low phosphorus)

2 tsp stevia powder

1 oz chopped almonds (low potassium)

1 tsp vanilla extract

1/2 tsp cinnamon

Fresh mint leaves for garnish

Instructions:

In a medium-sized bowl, combine the Greek yogurt, stevia powder, vanilla extract, and cinnamon. Mix well until the stevia is fully dissolved into the yogurt.

In serving glasses or bowls, start by layering a spoonful of the sweetened Greek yogurt mixture at the bottom.

Add a layer of sliced strawberries, followed by a layer of blueberries, and then a layer of raspberries.

Repeat the layers until the glasses are filled, finishing with a dollop of the sweetened Greek yogurt on top.

Sprinkle chopped almonds over the parfait for a delightful crunch.

Garnish each parfait with fresh mint leaves.

Chill in the refrigerator for at least 30 mins before serving to allow flavors to meld.

Nutrition (Per Serving): Calories 180 | Fat 6g | Carbs 20g | Protein 12g

2 tbsp erythritol (or other suitable sugar substitute)

Almond Crumble:

1 cup almond flour

2 tbsp unsalted butter, chilled and diced

2 tbsp erythritol

1/2 tsp ground cinnamon

Instructions:

Toss apples with butter, lemon juice, cinnamon, and sweetener. Top with crumble mixture. Bake at 350°F for 30 mins.

Nutrition (Per Serving): Calories 230 | Fat 15g | Carbs 22g | Protein 3g

88. Cinnamon Baked Apples with Almond Crumble

Preparation Time: 15 mins | Cooking Time: 30 mins | Serving Size: 4

Ingredients:

Ingredients:

4 large apples, cored and sliced

2 tbsp unsalted butter, melted

2 tbsp lemon juice

1 tsp ground cinnamon

89. Sugar-Free Lemon Chia Pudding

Preparation Time: 10 mins | Cooking Time: 0 mins | Serving Size: 2

Ingredients:

1.76 oz chia seeds

1 cup unsweetened almond milk

1 tbsp lemon zest

2 tbsp lemon juice

1/2 tsp vanilla extract

1-2 tbsp erythritol or sweetener of choice (adjust to taste)

Fresh berries for garnish (optional)

Instructions:

In a mixing bowl, combine the chia seeds, unsweetened almond milk, lemon zest, lemon juice, vanilla extract, and erythritol.

Whisk the ingredients together thoroughly to ensure the chia seeds are well distributed. Let the mixture sit for 5 mins.

After 5 mins, whisk the mixture again to prevent clumping. Cover the bowl and refrigerate for at least 2 hours or overnight.

Before serving, give the pudding a good stir to achieve a smooth consistency. If the pudding is too thick, you can add a little more almond milk until you reach your desired thickness.

Spoon the lemon chia pudding into serving glasses or bowls.

Garnish with fresh berries if desired.

Nutrition (Per serving): Calories 120 | Fat 7g | Carbs 12g | Protein 4g

90. Protein-Packed Greek Yogurt Berry Cups

Preparation Time: 10 mins | Cooking Time: 0 mins | Serving Size: 2

Ingredients:

Ingredients:

1 1/4 cups Greek yogurt (low phosphorus)

1 cup mixed berries

1/4 cup chopped almonds (low potassium)

2 tbsp chia seeds

1 tbsp honey (optional)

1 tsp vanilla extract

1 tsp lemon zest

Instructions:

Mix yogurt with vanilla and lemon zest. Layer yogurt, berries, almonds, and chia seeds in cups. Chill for 30 mins before serving.

Nutrition (Per Serving): Calories 250 | Fat 12g | Carbs 20g | Protein 15g

91. Warm Cinnamon Pear Compote

Preparation Time: 10 mins | Cooking Time: 20 mins | Serving Size: 4

Ingredients:

21.2 oz ripe pears, peeled, cored, and diced

1.76 oz granulated sugar substitute (suitable for renal diet)

1 tsp ground cinnamon

1/2 tsp vanilla extract

1/4 tsp ground nutmeg

1/2 cup water

1 tbsp lemon juice

Instructions:

In a medium-sized pot, combine the diced pears, sugar substitute, ground cinnamon, vanilla extract, ground nutmeg, water, and lemon juice.

Place the pot over medium heat and bring the mixture to a gentle boil.

Reduce the heat to low, cover the pot, and simmer for 15-20 mins or until the pears are tender. Stir occasionally to ensure even cooking.

Once the pears are soft and the mixture has thickened slightly, remove the pot from the heat.

Allow the compote to cool for a few mins before serving.

Serve the warm cinnamon pear compote on its own, over low-potassium ice cream or yogurt, or as a topping for a renal-friendly dessert.

Nutrition (Per Serving): Calories 80 | Fat 0g | Carbs 20g | Protein 0g

92. Baked Peach with Honey and Walnuts

Preparation Time: 15 mins | Cooking Time: 25 mins | Serving Size: 2

Ingredients:

4 ripe peaches (about 28 oz), halved and pitted

1/4 cup walnuts, chopped (consider a lower phosphorus alternative if needed)

2 tbsp honey (or suitable sugar substitute for renal diet)

2 tsp unsalted butter, melted

1 tsp cinnamon

1/2 tsp vanilla extract

Instructions:

Preheat the oven to 350°F (180°C).

Place peach halves, cut side up, in a baking dish.

In a bowl, mix walnuts, honey (or substitute), butter, cinnamon, and vanilla. Spoon over peaches.

Bake for 25 mins or until peaches are tender.

Serve warm, optionally with low-potassium ice cream or yogurt.

Nutrition (Per Serving): Calories 220 | Fat 10g | Carbs 30g | Protein 3g

93. Poached Apricots in Ginger Syrup

Preparation Time: 15 mins | Cooking Time: 10 mins | Serving Size: 4

Ingredients:

1.1 lb fresh apricots, halved and pitted

1 cup sugar substitute suitable for a renal diet

1 cup water

1 tbsp freshly grated ginger

1 tsp lemon zest

1 cinnamon stick

4 whole cloves

Instructions:

Combine sugar substitute, water, ginger, lemon zest, cinnamon, and cloves in a saucepan. Simmer until sugar dissolves.

Add apricots and poach for 5-7 mins until tender.

Let apricots cool in the syrup.

Serve chilled, drizzled with syrup.

Nutrition (Per serving): Calories 150 | Fat 0.5g | Carbs 38g | Protein 1g

94. Grilled Pineapple with Mint Drizzle

Preparation Time: 15 mins | Cooking Time: 8 mins | Serving Size: 4 persons

Ingredients:

21.2 oz fresh pineapple, peeled and sliced

0.35 oz fresh mint leaves, finely chopped

1 oz honey

1 tbsp lime juice

1 tsp olive oil

Instructions:

Preheat the grill to medium-high heat.

In a small bowl, mix together the honey, lime juice, and olive oil to create the drizzle sauce.

Place the pineapple slices on the preheated grill and cook for about 4 mins on each side, or until grill marks appear and the pineapple is slightly caramelized.

While the pineapple is grilling, prepare the mint drizzle. In a separate bowl, combine the finely chopped mint with the drizzle sauce mixture.

Once the pineapple slices are done grilling, remove them from the grill and arrange them on a serving platter.

Drizzle the mint sauce over the grilled pineapple slices.

Serve immediately and enjoy this refreshing and kidney-friendly dessert.

Nutrition (Per Serving): Calories 150 | Fat 3g | Carbs 35g | Protein 1g

95. Spiced Berry Medley with Citrus Glaze

Preparation Time: 15 mins | Cooking Time: 10 mins | Serving Size: 4 persons

Ingredients:

8.8 oz strawberries, hulled and halved

5.3 oz blueberries

3.5 oz raspberries

1.76 oz blackberries

2 tbsp honey

1 tsp ground cinnamon

1/2 tsp ground ginger

1/4 tsp ground nutmeg

Zest of 1 orange

Zest of 1 lemon

2 tbsp fresh orange juice

1 tbsp fresh lemon juice

Citrus Glaze:

2 tbsp honey

1 tbsp fresh orange juice

1 tsp cornstarch

Instructions:

Prepare the Berries:

In a large bowl, combine strawberries, blueberries, raspberries, and blackberries.

Spice it Up:

Add honey, ground cinnamon, ground ginger, ground nutmeg, orange zest, and lemon zest to the berries. Gently toss to coat evenly.

Citrus Boost:

In a small bowl, mix fresh orange juice and lemon juice. Pour over the spiced berries and toss again. Allow the berries to marinate for 10 mins.

Cooking Time:

In a non-stick skillet over medium heat, transfer the marinated berries. Cook for 5-7 mins, stirring occasionally, until the berries release their juices and become slightly tender.

Prepare the Glaze:

In a small saucepan, combine honey, fresh orange juice, and cornstarch. Cook over low heat, stirring continuously until the glaze thickens.

Final Touch:

Drizzle the citrus glaze over the cooked berries. Gently toss to coat. Remove from heat.

Serve:

Divide the spiced berry medley into four serving bowls. Garnish with additional citrus zest if desired.

Nutrition (Per Serving): Calories 120 | Fat 1g | Carbs 30g | Protein 1g

96. Creamy Avocado Lime Sorbet

Preparation Time: 10 mins | Cooking Time: 0 mins | Serving Size: 4

Ingredients:

14 oz ripe avocados, peeled and pitted

5 oz granulated sugar substitute (suitable for renal diet)

1 cup unsweetened almond milk (low in potassium)

1/4 cup lime juice

Zest of 2 limes

1 tsp vanilla extract

1/4 tsp salt

Instructions:

In a blender, combine the ripe avocados, sugar substitute, almond milk, lime juice, lime zest, vanilla extract, and salt.

Blend the ingredients until smooth and creamy.

Taste the mixture and adjust sweetness or tartness as needed by adding more sugar substitute or lime juice.

Pour the sorbet mixture into an ice cream maker and churn according to the manufacturer's instructions until it reaches a soft-serve consistency.

Transfer the sorbet to a lidded container and freeze for at least 4 hours or until firm.

Before serving, let the sorbet sit at room temperature for a few mins to soften slightly. Scoop the sorbet into bowls or cones and garnish with additional lime zest if desired.

Nutrition (Per serving): Calories 180 | Fat 11g | Carbs 20g | Protein 2g

97. Coconut Almond Bliss Ice Cream

Preparation Time: 10 mins | Cooking Time: 0 mins | Serving Size: 4

Ingredients:

14 oz coconut milk (unsweetened)

3.5 oz almonds, chopped

1.75 oz shredded coconut (unsweetened)

1.75 oz erythritol (or preferred sugar substitute)

1 tsp vanilla extract

1/4 tsp salt

Instructions:

In a blender, combine the coconut milk, chopped almonds, shredded coconut, erythritol, vanilla extract, and salt.

Blend until the mixture is smooth and well combined.

Pour the mixture into an ice cream maker and churn according to the manufacturer's instructions until it reaches a soft-serve consistency.

Transfer the churned ice cream into a lidded container and freeze for at least 4 hours or until firm.

Before serving, allow the ice cream to soften slightly at room temperature for easier scooping.

Serve the Coconut Almond Bliss Ice Cream in small portions.

Nutrition (Per Serving): Calories 250 | Fat 22g | Carbs 10g | Protein 5g

98. Mango Basil Sorbet with a Hint of Lime

Preparation Time: 15 mins | Cooking Time: 0 mins | Serving Size: 4

Ingredients:

1.3 lb ripe mango, peeled and diced

1/4 cup fresh basil leaves

Sugar substitute suitable for a renal diet, to taste

1/4 cup freshly squeezed lime juice

1 cup water

Instructions:

Blend mango, basil, sugar substitute, and lime juice until smooth.

Gradually add water and blend.

Churn in an ice cream maker or freeze, stirring occasionally.

Serve with additional basil or lime zest.

Nutrition (Per Serving): Calories: 267 | Fat: 19 g | Carbs: 12 g | Protein: 11 g

99. Vanilla Bean Frozen Yogurt Swirl

Preparation Time: 10 mins | Cooking Time: 0 mins | Serving Size: 4 persons

100. Berry Burst Sherbet with Fresh Mint

Preparation Time: 10 mins | Cooking Time: 0 mins | Serving Size: 4

Ingredients:

2 cups low-phosphorus Greek yogurt

Sugar substitute suitable for a renal diet, to taste

Seeds from 1 vanilla bean

1 tsp pure vanilla extract

Optional: 1/4 cup chopped fresh strawberries, for garnish

Optional: 2 tbsp chopped unsalted almonds, for garnish

Instructions:

Mix yogurt with sugar substitute, vanilla bean seeds, and extract.

Churn in an ice cream maker until soft-serve consistency.

Freeze until firm. Swirl in strawberries and almonds before serving.

Nutrition (Per Serving): Calories 120 | Fat 5g | Carbs 10g | Protein 10g

Ingredients:

1.1 lb mixed berries (strawberries, blueberries, raspberries)

Sugar substitute suitable for a renal diet, to taste

1 tbsp fresh lime juice

1/4 cup finely chopped fresh mint leaves

2 cups ice cubes

1 cup cold water

Instructions:

Blend berries, sugar substitute, lime juice, mint, and ice until smooth.

Add water and blend to desired consistency.

Serve immediately, garnished with mint leaves.

Nutrition (Per Serving): Calories 80 | Fat 0.5g | Carbs 20g | Protein 1g

Chapter 5: Managing Daily Challenges

Living with certain health conditions often requires a heightened awareness and careful management of daily challenges. For those navigating a renal diet, where the focus is on maintaining kidney health through mindful food choices, every day can present unique hurdles. However, with the right strategies and mindset, it is possible to overcome these challenges and lead a fulfilling and healthy life.

Tips for Eating Out While Maintaining a Renal Diet

Dining out can be both a pleasure and a challenge when following a renal diet. Here are some practical tips to help you enjoy restaurant meals while adhering to your dietary restrictions:

Research Beforehand: Check the restaurant's menu online before going out. This allows you to identify dishes that align with your renal diet, making it easier to make informed choices.

Communication is Key: Don't hesitate to communicate your dietary needs to the restaurant staff. Ask about ingredients, preparation methods, and possible substitutions to ensure your meal meets your specific requirements.

Choose Wisely: Opt for simple, grilled, or baked dishes rather than fried or heavily seasoned options. Lean proteins, such as chicken or fish, and a variety of fresh vegetables can be excellent choices.

Watch Portion Sizes: Restaurant portions are often larger than what you might eat at home. Consider sharing a dish with a dining companion or requesting a half portion to avoid overeating.

Be Mindful of Condiments: Sauces, dressings, and condiments can contribute to hidden sources of sodium and phosphorus. Ask for these on the side so you can control the amount you consume.

Stay Hydrated: Water is your best friend. Opt for water or other renal-friendly beverages instead of sugary or caffeinated options. Limiting your intake of sodas and alcohol is crucial for kidney health.

How to Handle Special Occasions and Holidays

Celebrations and special occasions often revolve around food, making it challenging to stick to a renal diet. Here's how you can navigate these events without compromising your health:

Plan Ahead: Anticipate the types of foods that may be served and plan your choices accordingly. If attending a potluck, consider bringing a renal-friendly dish to share.

Communicate with Hosts: Inform hosts of your dietary restrictions in advance. Most hosts appreciate knowing about specific needs and will often accommodate them.

Bring Your Own Dish: If you're unsure about the available food options, consider bringing a dish that aligns with your renal diet. This ensures you have a safe and enjoyable option.

Focus on Non-Food Activities: Shift the focus of the celebration away from food. Engage in activities, games, or conversations that don't revolve around eating, helping to de-emphasize the role of food in the event.

Practice Moderation: While it's okay to enjoy some special treats on occasion, moderation is key. Be mindful of portion sizes and try to balance indulgent foods with healthier choices.

Strategies to Stay Motivated and Adhere to the Diet

Maintaining motivation over the long term can be challenging, but it's crucial for the success of a renal diet. Consider these strategies to stay motivated and committed:

Set Realistic Goals: Break down your dietary goals into small, achievable steps. Celebrate your successes, no matter how minor, to stay motivated.

Educate Yourself: Learn more about the benefits of a renal diet and how it positively impacts kidney health. Understanding the "why" behind your dietary choices can reinforce your commitment.

Create a Support System: Share your dietary goals with friends, family, or a support group. Having a support system can provide encouragement, understanding, and accountability.

Reward Yourself: Establish a reward system for sticking to your renal diet. Treat yourself to non-food rewards, such as a relaxing day, a hobby you enjoy, or a small purchase when you achieve milestones.

Track Your Progress: Keep a food diary to monitor your dietary choices. This can help you identify patterns, make adjustments, and track your progress over time.

Celebrate Small Wins: Recognize and celebrate each successful day or week adhering to your renal diet. This positive reinforcement can help you stay motivated in the face of challenges.

By implementing these strategies, you can manage daily challenges, enjoy dining out, navigate special occasions, and stay motivated on your renal diet journey. Remember that consistency and a positive mindset are key components of long-term success.

Chapter 6: Adapting the Renal Diet to Individual Needs

The journey to maintaining kidney health is not a one-size-fits-all approach. As we delve into the intricacies of the renal diet, it becomes evident that customization is key to its success. Adapting the renal diet to individual needs involves tailoring nutritional plans to accommodate specific health conditions, lifestyles, and dietary preferences. In this chapter, we will explore the importance of customization and provide practical guidance on how to modify the renal diet to suit different individuals.

Customizing the Diet According to One's Health Conditions

Individuals grappling with kidney-related issues often have diverse health conditions that need careful consideration. The renal diet, while primarily focused on managing kidney function, can be adapted to address concurrent health challenges. For example, those with cardiovascular issues may need to incorporate heart-healthy elements into their renal diet, such as incorporating omega-3 fatty acids and minimizing sodium intake.

Patients with diabetes face a unique set of challenges as diabetes and kidney disease often go hand in hand. Balancing blood sugar levels becomes paramount. This leads us to our next point.

Special Considerations for Diabetics and Hypertensive Individuals

For individuals managing both kidney disease and diabetes, achieving glycemic control is crucial. The renal diet for diabetics should not only monitor phosphorus and potassium but also carefully manage carbohydrates. Selecting complex carbohydrates over simple sugars can aid in stabilizing blood glucose levels.

Hypertension, or high blood pressure, is another common companion to kidney disease. Reducing sodium intake is vital for hypertensive individuals. Hence, a dual focus on both potassium and sodium becomes pivotal in crafting a diet that caters to the intricacies of renal health and blood pressure management.

By collaborating with healthcare professionals, individuals can create a personalized renal diet plan that effectively addresses these coexisting health conditions.

Advice for Vegetarians and Vegans

Dietary preferences, such as following a vegetarian or vegan lifestyle, add an extra layer of complexity to the renal diet. Navigating protein sources, typically abundant in meat, requires careful planning for plant-based enthusiasts. Fortunately, various plant-based protein options exist, such as legumes, tofu, and certain grains.

Vegetarians and vegans must pay special attention to nutrient absorption and ensure they obtain essential vitamins and minerals from alternative sources. Calcium, iron, and vitamin B12, for instance, may need supplementation or strategic food choices.

In summary, adapting the renal diet to individual needs involves a comprehensive approach that incorporates considerations for diverse health conditions, special attention to diabetics and hypertensive individuals, and thoughtful advice for vegetarians and vegans. By tailoring the renal diet to suit individual circumstances, individuals can strike a balance that supports kidney health while aligning with their unique health profiles and preferences.

Chapter 7: FAQ - Frequently Asked Questions about the Renal Diet.

The renal diet is a crucial component of managing kidney health. As individuals navigate the complexities of dietary restrictions to support kidney function, it's common to have questions. In this chapter, we'll address some of the frequently asked questions about the renal diet to provide clarity and guidance.

1. Why is a Renal Diet Necessary?

The renal diet is essential for individuals with kidney disease because it helps manage the levels of certain nutrients in the body, such as sodium, potassium, and phosphorus. By controlling these elements, the diet helps reduce the strain on the kidneys and minimizes the risk of complications associated with kidney dysfunction.

2. What Foods Should I Limit on a Renal Diet?

Certain foods are restricted in a renal diet to avoid overloading the kidneys. Common restrictions include foods high in sodium, potassium, and phosphorus. This often involves limiting the intake of processed foods, canned goods, high-potassium fruits and vegetables, and dairy products.

3. How Can I Manage Protein Intake in a Renal Diet?

Protein is a crucial nutrient, but excessive protein intake can be harmful to the kidneys. Individuals on a renal diet should work with their healthcare team to determine an appropriate level of protein intake. High-quality protein sources such as lean meats, poultry, fish, and eggs are preferred, and portion control is emphasized.

4. Is Fluid Intake Important in a Renal Diet?

Yes, managing fluid intake is vital in a renal diet. Individuals with kidney disease may experience fluid retention, leading to swelling and increased blood pressure. Monitoring and restricting fluid intake help manage these symptoms. The recommended fluid intake can vary based on individual health conditions, so it's essential to consult with a healthcare professional.

5. Can I Still Enjoy Flavorful Meals on a Renal Diet?

Absolutely! While there are restrictions, a renal diet can still be diverse and flavorful. Herbs, spices, and other low-sodium seasonings can add taste to meals without compromising kidney health. Experimenting with different cooking methods, such as grilling, baking, or roasting, can enhance the flavor of foods without relying on excessive salt.

6. How Does a Renal Diet Impact Bone Health?

Phosphorus regulation is crucial for maintaining bone health in individuals with kidney disease. The renal diet aims to control phosphorus levels, often by limiting the consumption of phosphorus-rich foods like dairy products and certain meats. Calcium supplements may be recommended to help balance calcium and phosphorus levels.

7. Can I Follow a Vegetarian or Vegan Renal Diet?

Yes, it is possible to follow a vegetarian or vegan renal diet with careful planning. Plant-based protein sources such as beans, lentils, and tofu can be included, but individuals need to pay close attention to potassium and phosphorus levels in plant-based foods. Consulting with a registered dietitian is essential for creating a well-balanced and personalized vegetarian or vegan renal diet plan.

8. How Often Should I Monitor My Blood Values?

Monitoring blood values is crucial for individuals with kidney disease. The frequency of blood tests may vary based on the stage of kidney disease and individual health needs. Regular check-ups with healthcare providers help track changes in kidney function, electrolyte levels, and other essential parameters, allowing for timely adjustments to the renal diet plan.

9. Are Cheat Days Allowed on a Renal Diet?

Cheat days or occasional indulgences may be possible, but they should be approached with caution. It's essential to discuss any deviations from the renal diet with healthcare providers, as sudden changes in nutrient intake can impact kidney function. Moderation and communication with the healthcare team are key when considering occasional treats.

10. Can I Travel While Following a Renal Diet?

Yes, it is possible to travel while following a renal diet. Planning ahead is crucial, and individuals should be prepared with suitable snacks, a list of renal-friendly restaurants, and any necessary medical documentation for medications or dietary needs. Staying hydrated during travel is also important, so it's essential to carry an adequate supply of water.

In conclusion, the renal diet is a nuanced and individualized approach to managing kidney health. While it comes with certain restrictions, it is possible to maintain a satisfying and diverse diet with careful planning and guidance from healthcare professionals. Regular communication with a healthcare team ensures that the renal diet is tailored to meet individual needs and supports overall well-being.

30 - Day Meal Plan

Days	Breakfast	Lunch	Dinner	Snacks/Desserts
1	Quick Berry Blast Smoothie	Quinoa and Veggie Delight Salad	Grilled Lemon Herb Salmon with Quinoa	Savory Chickpea Delight
2	Easy Banana Almond Porridge	Grilled Chicken Caesar Salad	Baked Rosemary Chicken Breast with Vegetables	Crispy Kale Chips
3	Protein-Packed Spinach Omelette	Spinach and Berry Power Salad	Garlic Parmesan Crusted Tilapia	Zesty Guacamole Bruschetta
4	Wholesome Blueberry Pancakes	Mediterranean Chickpea Salad Bowl	Lemon Dill Grilled Chicken Skewers	Spicy Roasted Edamame
5	Speedy Mango Tango Smoothie	Roasted Beet and Goat Cheese Salad	Spicy Blackened Cod with Roasted Asparagus	Tomato Basil Quinoa Bites
6	Simple Cinnamon Apple Porridge	Avocado and Shrimp Citrus Salad	Pesto Baked Chicken Thighs with Green Beans	Tropical Paradise Parfait
7	High-Protein Veggie Omelette Cups	Cucumber and Dill Yogurt Salad	Teriyaki Glazed Salmon with Brown Rice	Berries and Cream Delight
8	Nutty Banana Walnut Muffins	Watermelon and Feta Summer Salad	Mediterranean Herb Crusted Snapper	Mango Tango Smoothie Bowl
9	Refreshing Green Smoothie	Broccoli and Cranberry Almond Salad	Cilantro Lime Grilled Chicken with Zucchini Noodles	Pineapple Coconut Yogurt Popsicles
10	Creamy Coconut Chia Porridge	Tuna and White Bean Mediterranean Salad	Baked Herb-Crusted Haddock with Cauliflower Mash	Citrus Burst Fruit Salad
11	Lean Turkey and Veggie Omelette	Lemon Herb Chicken Soup with Brown Rice	Chickpea and Spinach Curry	Nutty Banana Oat Bars

Days	Breakfast	Lunch	Dinner	Snacks/Desserts
12	Quinoa Pancakes with Mixed Berries	Vegetable and Lentil Broth with Fresh Herbs	Black Bean and Quinoa Stuffed Peppers	Cranberry Almond Energy Bites
13	Breezy Tropical Smoothie Bowl	Butternut Squash and Apple Soup	Creamy Tuscan White Bean Pasta	Date and Walnut Bliss Balls
14	Five-Minute Chocolate Oat Porridge	Turkey and Vegetable Quinoa Chowder	Sweet Potato and Chickpea Buddha Bowl	Chia Seed Pudding Parfait
15	Zesty Tomato and Feta Omelette	Creamy Cauliflower and Leek Soup	Red Lentil Dal with Coconut Milk	Blueberry Quinoa Bars
16	Gluten-Free Blueberry Muffins	Turkey and Cranberry Wrap with Spinach	Mediterranean Three-Bean Salad	Guilt-Free Chocolate Avocado Mousse
17	Protein-Packed Peanut Butter Smoothie	Grilled Salmon and Avocado Whole Grain Wrap	Spicy Black Bean and Corn Quesadillas	Stevia-Sweetened Berry Parfait
18	Easy Apple Cinnamon Pancakes	Egg Salad Lettuce Wraps with Fresh Herbs	Quinoa and Black-Eyed Pea Salad	Cinnamon Baked Apples with Almond Crumble
19	Spinach and Mushroom Egg White Omelette	Mediterranean Hummus and Veggie Sandwich	Eggplant and Lentil Moussaka	Sugar-Free Lemon Chia Pudding
20	Sweet Potato Pancakes with Maple Pecan Glaze	Chicken and Pesto Caprese Panini with Low-Phosphorus Bread	Lentil and Vegetable Stew	Protein-Packed Greek Yogurt Berry Cups
21	Quinoa Pancakes with Mixed Berries	Grilled Salmon and Avocado Whole Grain Wrap	Lemon Herb Baked Cod with Couscous	Warm Cinnamon Pear Compote
22	Breezy Tropical Smoothie Bowl	Egg Salad Lettuce Wraps with Fresh Herbs	Cheesy Broccoli and Chicken Casserole	Poached Apricots in Ginger Syrup
23	Five-Minute Chocolate Oat Porridge	Mediterranean Hummus and Veggie Sandwich	Creamy Tomato Basil Risotto with Grilled Chicken	Grilled Pineapple with Mint Drizzle

Days	Breakfast	Lunch	Dinner	Snacks/Desserts
24	Zesty Tomato and Feta Omelette	Chicken and Pesto Caprese Panini with Low-Phosphorus Bread	Spinach and Feta Stuffed Portobello Mushrooms	Spiced Berry Medley with Citrus Glaze
25	Gluten-Free Blueberry Muffins	Grilled Salmon and Avocado Whole Grain Wrap	Mexican Quinoa Casserole with Black Beans	Creamy Avocado Lime Sorbet
26	Protein-Packed Peanut Butter Smoothie	Egg Salad Lettuce Wraps with Fresh Herbs	Lemon Garlic Shrimp and Rice Skillet	Coconut Almond Bliss Ice Cream
27	Easy Apple Cinnamon Pancakes	Mediterranean Hummus and Veggie Sandwich	Sweet Potato and Kale Frittata	Mango Basil Sorbet with a Hint of Lime
28	Spinach and Mushroom Egg White Omelette	Chicken and Pesto Caprese Panini with Low-Phosphorus Bread	Creamy Tuscan White Bean Pasta	Vanilla Bean Frozen Yogurt Swirl
29	Sweet Potato Pancakes with Maple Pecan Glaze	Grilled Salmon and Avocado Whole Grain Wrap	Spinach and Feta Stuffed Portobello Mushrooms	Berry Burst Sherbet with Fresh Mint
30	Quinoa Pancakes with Mixed Berries	Egg Salad Lettuce Wraps with Fresh Herbs	Mexican Quinoa Casserole with Black Beans	Coconut Almond Bliss Ice Cream

Feel free to adjust the plan to suit your preferences and dietary needs. Enjoy your meals!

Measurement Conversion Table

VOLUME EQUIVALENTS (LIQUID)

US STANDARD	US STANDARD (OUNCES)	METRIC (APPROXIMATE)
2 tablespoons	1 fl. oz.	30 mL
1/4 cup	2 fl. oz.	60 mL
1/2 cup	4 fl. oz.	120 mL
1 cup	8 fl. oz.	240 mL
1-1/2 cups	12 fl. oz.	355 mL
2 cups or 1 pint	16 fl. oz.	475 mL
4 cups or 1 quart	32 fl. oz.	1 L
1 gallon	128 fl. oz.	4 L

VOLUME EQUIVALENTS (DRY)

US STANDARD	METRIC (APPROXIMATE)
1/8 teaspoon	0.5 mL
1/4 teaspoon	1 mL
1/2 teaspoon	2 mL
3/4 teaspoon	4 mL
1 teaspoon	5 mL
1 tablespoon	15 mL
1/4 cup	59 mL
1/3 cup	79 mL

1/2 cup	118 mL
2/3 cup	156 mL
3/4 cup	177 mL
1 cup	235 mL
2 cups	475 mL
3 cups	700 mL
4 cups	1 L

OVEN TEMPERATURES

FAHRENHEIT (F)	CELSIUS (C) (APPROXIMATE)
250°	120°
300°	150°
325°	165°
350°	180°
375°	190°
400°	200°
425°	220°
450°	230°

WEIGHT EQUIVALENTS

US STANDARD	METRIC (APPROXIMATE)
1/2 ounce	15 g
1 ounce	30 g
2 ounces	60 g
4 ounces	115 g
8 ounces	225 g
12 ounces	340 g
16 ounces or 1 pound	455 g

Conclusion

In concluding this Renal Diet Cookbook for Beginners, we hope that you have found not only a collection of delicious recipes but also a valuable resource for managing a renal-friendly lifestyle. The journey toward better kidney health is a continuous one, and your commitment to making positive dietary choices is a commendable step in the right direction.

By embracing the principles of a renal diet, you have empowered yourself with the knowledge to support your kidneys and enhance overall well-being. Remember, this cookbook is just the beginning of your culinary exploration within the realm of renal-friendly meals. Feel free to experiment with the recipes, tweak them to suit your taste preferences, and discover new flavors that align with your dietary needs.

As you embark on this journey, continue to consult with healthcare professionals to ensure that your dietary choices align with your unique health circumstances. Consistency and moderation are key, and by incorporating the principles of a renal diet into your daily routine, you are taking proactive steps toward maintaining optimal kidney function.

We hope this cookbook has not only provided you with nourishing recipes but also inspired a greater appreciation for the connection between food and health. May your kitchen be a place of creativity, wellness, and joy as you savor each bite on your renal diet journey.

Here's to your health and the flavorful chapters that lie ahead in your culinary adventure!

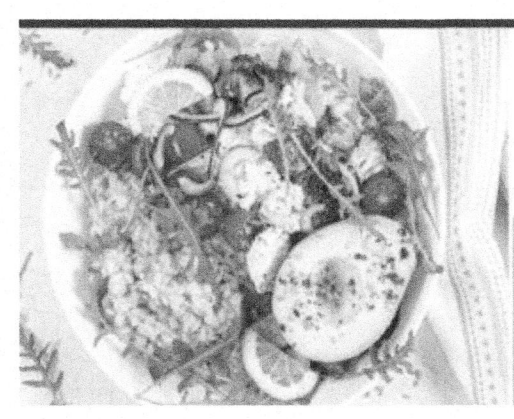

SCANNING THE QR CODE

OR COPY THE LINK TO DOWNLOAD THE BONUS

https://2ly.link/1ws6l

Made in the USA
Monee, IL
28 July 2025

22099720R00070